THE CRAP WE CONSUME

BY UMESH M PHERWANI

Umesh Pherwani is a life coach a NLP trainer and a keynote speaker.His first book 'Are you out of your mind' was very well received and marked his first steps into the literary world.
Born in Mumbai, he completed his Masters in Psychology and is pursuing a Ph.D. in the same line of study. Umesh completed a 125 hours program in neuroscience and the neurobiology of behavior from Stanford university.
His second book was The Mind Switch which was the first in the trio series, followed by The Body Switch and The Gut Switch.

Umesh M Pherwani
www.umeshpherwani.com

Dedication

To my dad with everlasting love and gratitude

PROLOGUE

Prologue: Unveiling the Crap We Consume

In a world bustling with choices and temptations, we find ourselves at a pivotal juncture – a crossroads where indulgence and insight collide. Our journey through the labyrinth of modern consumption begins with a single question: What have we been feeding ourselves?

Welcome to a voyage of discovery, an odyssey into the heart of our culinary choices and dietary habits. This is not a tale of judgment, but an exploration – a quest to uncover the layers of convenience, marketing, and subconscious yearnings that shape the world of "The Crap We Consume."

In the era of fast-paced lives and frenzied schedules, we've become adept at navigating the shelves of supermarkets, deciphering nutritional labels, and decoding food trends. Yet, amidst the sea of products promising convenience, taste, and satisfaction, a deeper truth lurks beneath the surface. We've unknowingly surrendered a portion of our well-being to a cacophony of processed temptations, sugar-laden delights, and convenient concoctions.

This prologue is our call to arms – a clarion to awaken our senses and reclaim our agency over the choices that grace our plates. As we traverse the landscapes of fast food frenzies, delve into the science of cravings, and unravel the intricacies of food marketing, we are confronted with the undeniable reality: the crap we consume is more than just a matter of sustenance – it is a reflection of our culture, desires, and the intricate dance between pleasure and responsibility.

As we embark on this eye-opening journey, we must brace ourselves for revelations that challenge our assumptions, provoke self-reflection, and ignite a desire for change. We'll encounter tales of indulgence and redemption, stories of transformation and triumph, and dive deep into the underbelly of the food industry that seeks to tantalize our senses and hijack our cravings.

Yet, this is not a tale of despair, but a narrative of empowerment. Through knowledge and understanding, we forge a path toward mindful consumption and informed decisions. Together, we shall shed the shroud of ignorance and emerge as stewards of our well-being, guardians of our health, and champions of conscious choices.

So, dear reader, let us set forth on this remarkable expedition – a journey that promises to illuminate the shadows of our dietary habits, challenge our notions of what we consume, and unveil the secrets behind "The Crap We Consume." As we turn the pages, we are invited to embrace a new perspective, an enlightened relationship with food, and the power to reshape our culinary destinies. The voyage has begun; may it be one of enlightenment, transformation, and culinary liberation.

1. INTRODUCTION
UNRAVELING THE TEMPTING TAPESTRY

Welcome to a world where the delectable dance of flavors meets the mysterious realm of indulgence. A world where convenience beckons, and taste triumphs over reason. This, dear reader, is the realm of junk food – a tantalizing tapestry woven from the threads of guilty pleasures, culinary adventures, and the undeniable allure of the forbidden.

In this journey through the pages ahead, we shall embark on a quest to uncover the hidden stories, peculiar histories, and quirky truths behind the foods we love to hate and hate to love. Yes, we're diving headfirst into the realm of processed, packaged, and palate-pleasing delights that we affectionately

– and sometimes begrudgingly – refer to as "junk food."

But what exactly is junk food, you might wonder? Is it just an arbitrary label slapped onto snacks and treats that might not fit the conventional definition of healthy eating? Or does it carry a deeper, more complex significance in the modern gastronomic landscape?

Buckle up, because we're about to explore this intricate gastronomic universe. From the initial sizzle of French fries meeting hot oil to the satisfying crunch of a perfectly coated potato chip, from the nostalgia of a candy bar wrapper to the fleeting satisfaction of an impulse buy at the supermarket checkout line – we'll uncover the psychology, history, and even the science that drives our insatiable appetite for these culinary guilty pleasures.

But this isn't just a journey of culinary curiosity; it's a quest to understand our relationship with the foods that simultaneously entice and perplex us. We'll peel back the layers of marketing magic that make us crave certain items and examine the underlying emotions that lead us to turn to junk food in times of both celebration and despair.

With each chapter, we'll reveal the complex interplay between taste and health, desire and discipline, and culture and commerce. We'll laugh at our shared quirks, gasp at the shocking revelations, and nod in recognition as we discover the absurd yet irresistible connections that make up the story of junk food.

So, let's put on our detective hats and embark on this flavorful expedition. From drive-thru windows to late-night snacking escapades, from supersized meals to minuscule candies, we'll uncover the secrets, expose the myths, and ultimately answer the question that lingers in the back of our minds: What truly lies behind the captivating allure of the crap we consume?

2.
UNRAVELING THE JUNK FOOD MYTH: WHAT REALLY LIES BENEATH

In a world saturated with culinary choices, where farm-to-table feasts and organic indulgences reign supreme, there exists a peculiar, often misunderstood category of sustenance: junk food. These bite-sized morsels of pleasure, wrapped in vibrant packaging and adorned with promises of instant gratification, have sparked a cultural phenomenon that has left no corner of the globe untouched. From the neon-lit streets of bustling metropolises to the quiet, tree-lined avenues of suburbia, junk food has woven its way into the fabric of our lives, forging a love affair that is as puzzling as it is undeniable.

But what exactly is junk food? Is it merely the sum of its empty calories and questionable ingredients, or does it possess a deeper significance that eludes the casual observer? In this chapter, we embark on a journey to unravel the layers of the junk food myth, peering beyond the surface to discover the intricate web of psychology, history, and culture that underlies our collective obsession with these tantalizing treats.

The Origins of Indulgence

To understand the present, we must delve into the past. The roots of junk food trace back through centuries of culinary evolution, mingling with historical shifts in societal norms, technological advancements, and economic changes. The concept of indulgence, of savoring delectable flavors without concern for nutritional value, is not a recent invention. Our ancestors reveled in honey-drenched confections and lavish feasts long before the modern convenience store emerged.

However, the dawn of the Industrial Revolution in the late 18th century marked a turning point in the way we approached food. As urbanization surged, and factory jobs replaced traditional agricultural lifestyles, people's dietary habits shifted. Processed foods emerged as a means of providing sustenance to the masses, giving rise to canned goods, preserved meats, and early incarnations of what we now know as snack foods.

From Cornflakes to Cheetos: The Rise of Convenience

The early 20th century witnessed a proliferation of ready-to-eat options that catered to the fast-paced lifestyle of the modern urban dweller. In an era of innovation, breakfast cereals like Cornflakes promised health and convenience in a box. Meanwhile, the creation of the potato chip, often attributed to a fateful day in 1853 when chef George Crum sliced potatoes paper-thin in a fit of frustration, laid the foundation for the snack food industry.

The mid-20th century saw the birth of iconic fast food chains like McDonald's, Burger King, and KFC, transforming the act of dining out into a standardized, mass-produced experience. The expansion of suburbs and the rise of the automobile culture further fueled the demand for quick, on-the-go sustenance.

The Psychology of Cravings

Junk food's allure extends beyond mere convenience. It taps into our primal instincts, triggering a cascade of sensory experiences that hijack our senses and leave us craving more. The perfect crunch of a chip, the melt-in-your-mouth creaminess of chocolate, and the satisfying burst of flavor from a savory snack – these sensations are meticulously engineered to provide instant gratification and create a cycle of reward that keeps us coming back for more.

Marketing plays a crucial role in amplifying these sensory triggers. Clever packaging, vibrant colors, and strategic placement in stores all contribute to the illusion of desirability. Furthermore, the psychology of scarcity and indulgence comes into play. The limited-time offers, seasonal treats, and promotional tie-ins capitalize on our fear of missing out, driving us to indulge in the fleeting pleasure of a forbidden delicacy.

Behind the Ingredients Curtain

Peering beneath the surface of a bag of chips or a candy bar unveils a world of ingredients that often defy comprehension. Hydrogenated oils, high fructose corn syrup, artificial flavors, and a laundry list of unpronounceable additives are the building blocks of many junk food items. These components, designed to enhance shelf life, texture, and taste, often contribute to the perceived 'addictiveness' of junk food, triggering our brain's pleasure centers in ways that echo the effects of drugs.

Moreover, the carefully calibrated balance of sweet, salty, and umami flavors in these foods can overwhelm our taste buds, making it harder to savor more subtle, natural tastes. This phenomenon is often referred to as "flavor fatigue," a state in which our palate becomes accustomed to intense flavors, leading us to seek out even more extreme tastes to achieve the same level of satisfaction.

The Culture of Crap

As junk food evolved, it insinuated itself into the cultural zeitgeist, becoming a symbol of leisure, indulgence, and even rebellion. Movie nights, road trips, and parties are incomplete without a selection of junk food delights. Iconic brand mascots, like the cheerful M&M characters or the mischievous Pringles can, have become pop culture icons, further cementing the association between junk food and carefree enjoyment.

Yet, this cultural fascination has not been without controversy. The rise of junk food has led to concerns about public health, as rates of obesity, diabetes, and other diet-related diseases have surged. The paradox of indulgence versus responsibility fuels debates about personal choice, societal influence, and the role of government in regulating food industries.

Conclusion

As we peel back the layers of the junk food myth, we uncover a complex tapestry of history, psychology, and culture that shapes our relationship with these delectable yet dubious treats. From their humble origins to their starring role in modern food culture, junk food items are more than the sum of their ingredients. They are cultural touchstones, emotional triggers, and sensory symphonies that resonate deep within our collective psyche.

In the chapters that follow, we will delve even deeper into the heart of this phenomenon, exploring the emotional roller coaster of indulgence, examining the surprising science of cravings, and unraveling the impact of junk food on our health, economy, and environment. So, dear reader, fasten your seatbelt and prepare for a journey through the delectable labyrinth of junk food – a journey that will challenge your perceptions, tickle your taste buds, and perhaps leave you questioning what really lies beneath the wrappers of the crap we consume.

3.
THE ALLURE OF EMPTY CALORIES: WHY WE CAN'T RESIST

In the ever-evolving landscape of gastronomy, where culinary innovation and health-conscious choices intertwine, one question persists: Why do we find it so difficult to resist the siren call of junk food? From crispy potato chips to sugary confections, the allure of empty calories beckons us, and we often find ourselves unable to resist their tantalizing embrace. In this chapter, we delve into the multifaceted reasons behind our persistent cravings for junk food, exploring the intricate interplay of biology, psychology, and societal factors that drive our insatiable appetite for indulgence.

The Pleasure Principle

At the heart of our fascination with junk food lies an intricate dance between our brain's reward system and the hedonistic pleasure it bestows. Foods high in fat, sugar, and salt activate the brain's release of dopamine, often referred to as the "feel-good" neurotransmitter. This biochemical reaction creates a sense of euphoria and satisfaction, effectively conditioning us to associate these foods with pleasure.

This pleasurable response is deeply rooted in our evolutionary history. Our ancestors, who relied on hunting and gathering, were naturally inclined to seek out energy-dense foods to ensure survival during times of scarcity. In the modern era of abundance, however, this primal instinct becomes a double-edged sword. The same mechanism that once safeguarded our survival now contributes to overconsumption and the allure of calorie-rich, nutrient-poor fare.

The Flavor Equation

Junk food's appeal extends beyond the physiological realm to the realm of the senses. The carefully crafted combination of flavors and textures in these items engages our taste buds in a symphony of sensations. The perfect balance of sweet, salty, and savory flavors, often accompanied by a satisfying crunch or melt-in-your-mouth creaminess, creates a sensory experience that is nothing short of irresistible.

Food scientists, armed with an arsenal of research and cutting-edge technology, meticulously engineer these flavors to optimize our sensory pleasure. It's not just the taste that matters; it's the way it feels, sounds, and even looks. The mere thought of sinking your teeth into a crispy chip or savoring the smoothness of chocolate can trigger anticipatory pleasure that primes your brain for indulgence.

The Emotional Connection

Junk food's appeal goes beyond the realm of the physical and sensory – it also taps into the emotional contours of our lives. Comfort, nostalgia, celebration, and even rebellion are often intertwined with our consumption of these foods. We associate them with moments of joy, relief, and camaraderie, imbuing them with a sense of emotional significance that transcends their nutritional value.

During times of stress or emotional turmoil, many of us turn to junk food as a form of solace. The familiar taste and texture offer a sense of security and comfort, momentarily alleviating our worries. Moreover, the act of indulgence itself can be a rebellion against dietary restrictions or societal norms, a small act of defiance that allows us to assert our autonomy and indulge in a guilty pleasure.

The Power of Advertising

The allure of junk food is amplified by the art of marketing – a craft that weaves desire and fantasy into the very fabric of our culture. Advertisements often portray these foods as gateways to happiness, adventure, and social connection. The glossy images of perfectly arranged burgers, colorful candies, and cascading soda bubbles tap into our aspirations, promising a brief escape from the mundane.

Furthermore, advertising leverages the psychology of visual cues and brand recognition to establish deep-rooted associations. Iconic logos, catchy slogans, and recognizable packaging create a sense of familiarity that makes these products almost comforting, like old friends waiting to offer a moment of pleasure.

The Social Context

Junk food's allure is not confined to personal cravings; it extends to the social fabric of our lives. Sharing a pizza during a movie night, passing around a bag of chips at a gathering, or treating oneself to a dessert after a meal are all rituals that foster connection and camaraderie. These shared experiences build bonds and memories, enhancing the emotional value of junk food.

Moreover, the ubiquity of junk food in our social interactions makes it a norm rather than an exception. It becomes a default choice when faced with time constraints or a lack of alternatives. The fast-paced nature of modern life often pushes us to prioritize convenience, and junk food offers a quick solution that fits seamlessly into our hectic routines.

The Paradox of Choice

While the allure of junk food may seem straightforward, the paradox of choice adds a layer of complexity to our cravings. In a world brimming with options, our brains often default to familiar choices – the ones that have consistently provided pleasure in the past. This phenomenon, known as decision fatigue, can lead us to opt for the tried-and-true comforts of junk food rather than navigating the overwhelming array of healthier alternatives.

Additionally, the perceived convenience of junk food plays a role in this decision-making process. The act of making multiple choices can feel mentally taxing, and junk food offers a reprieve from this cognitive burden. It becomes the default choice, the path of least resistance that requires minimal thought or effort.

Conclusion

The allure of empty calories, the siren call of junk food, is a symphony of biological responses, sensory indulgence, emotional connections, and societal influences. It's a dance between pleasure and desire, a delicate balance between the immediate gratification of our senses and the long-term considerations of our health.

In the chapters ahead, we will delve even deeper into the fascinating world of junk food psychology. We will explore the concept of emotional eating, dissect the mechanics of food addiction, and investigate the role of marketing in shaping our desires. As we unravel the intricate threads of our relationship with junk food, we will gain insight into the mechanisms that drive our cravings and the strategies that can empower us to make more mindful choices. So, dear reader, join us on this journey as we peel back the layers of temptation and examine the complex allure of empty calories that leaves us yearning for more.

4.

GUILTY PLEASURES AND MIDNIGHT MUNCHIES: CONFESSIONS OF A JUNK FOOD JUNKIE

Picture this: It's the dead of night, the world outside is hushed in slumber, and you find yourself sneaking into the kitchen. The glow of the refrigerator or the pantry's dim light beckons, and you're on a mission. Your heart races as you reach for that familiar bag of chips, that hidden stash of chocolate, or that container of cookies. Guilty pleasures come alive in the darkness, and you are not alone. In this chapter, we delve into the world of guilty pleasures and midnight munchies, exploring the hidden corners of our relationship with junk food and the often-secret rituals that define our indulgence.

The Dance of Temptation

There's a certain allure to indulging in guilty pleasures – the thrill of secrecy, the rebellion against societal norms, and the taste of forbidden fruit. It's as if junk food transforms into a partner in crime, a companion who understands and indulges our desires. In these moments of indulgence, we temporarily shed the burdens of responsibility and savor the pleasure that comes with succumbing to our cravings.

These secret escapades are not just about satisfying hunger; they're about fulfilling emotional needs. The act of giving in to a craving, of treating oneself, can provide a sense of comfort and relief from stress or emotional turmoil. In a world filled with demands and pressures, junk food becomes a brief respite, a guilty pleasure that momentarily silences the chaos.

The Comfort of Familiarity

The allure of junk food is often intertwined with nostalgia – a yearning for the tastes and textures of yesteryears. Childhood memories of after-school snacks, birthday parties, and summer treats are etched in our minds, creating a powerful emotional connection to certain foods. When the world feels overwhelming, these comfort foods offer a soothing balm, transporting us to simpler times.

The familiar crunch of a chip or the creamy sweetness of a candy bar triggers a rush of memories and emotions. It's a culinary time machine that allows us to relive moments of joy and innocence. As a result, junk food becomes more than just sustenance; it becomes a portal to cherished memories, a taste of the past that provides solace in the present.

The Pleasure of Ritual

Midnight munchies and secret snacking often involve a ritualistic dance – a series of steps that build anticipation and heighten the experience. From selecting the perfect snack to finding the right spot for indulgence, these rituals are deeply ingrained in the act of indulgence itself. The very process of unwrapping a candy bar or arranging a plate of treats becomes a sensory experience that amplifies the pleasure.

Furthermore, these rituals can be a form of self-care, a deliberate act of treating oneself to a moment of indulgence and pleasure. The act of creating a cozy setting, dimming the lights, and savoring each bite can transform a mundane activity into a sensory celebration, elevating the experience from mere consumption to a ritual of self-love.

The Theater of Taste

Junk food's appeal goes beyond flavor; it's also about the theater of taste. Think about the satisfying crackle of a chip, the gradual melting of chocolate on your tongue, or the delightful fizz of a carbonated beverage. These sensory experiences engage not only our taste buds but also our other senses, creating a multisensory symphony that captivates our attention and heightens our enjoyment.

Moreover, the act of eating junk food can be an immersive experience, a temporary escape from reality. The pleasure derived from each bite distracts us from our worries, enveloping us in a cocoon of sensory delight. It's a momentary escape from the demands of the day, a brief interlude where we can lose ourselves in the flavors and textures that titillate our senses.

Conquering Guilt: The Battle of Mind and Palate

As much as we relish the joys of indulgence, guilt often follows closely on its heels. The clash between the instant gratification of indulgence and the lingering awareness of its potential consequences can create a complex emotional landscape. Guilt, shame, and self-criticism can arise as we grapple with the aftermath of our cravings.

Navigating this emotional terrain requires a delicate balance – one that acknowledges the pleasure of indulgence while also recognizing the importance of mindful choices. Learning to enjoy guilty pleasures without succumbing to guilt is a journey of self-discovery and self-compassion. It involves cultivating a healthier relationship with food, one that allows for occasional indulgence without sacrificing overall well-being.

Conclusion

Guilty pleasures and midnight munchies reveal the intimate dance between our desires, emotions, and senses. They offer a glimpse into the often-hidden rituals that define our relationship with junk food, and the emotional nuances that underlie our indulgence. In these moments of secrecy and sensory delight, we find both solace and complexity – a reflection of our humanity and our quest for balance.

In the chapters that follow, we will dive deeper into the psychology of emotional eating, explore strategies to navigate cravings, and unveil the surprising ways in which junk food impacts our emotional well-being. As we continue our journey through the intricate world of junk food, we'll uncover the mechanisms that drive our behavior and gain insights into how we can cultivate a more mindful and empowered approach to our culinary desires. So, dear reader, join us as we peel back the layers of our midnight confessions and explore the complex tapestry of guilt and pleasure that defines our journey as junk food junkies.

5.

THE SWEET SEDUCTION: SUGAR'S ROLE IN OUR LOVE AFFAIR WITH JUNK

Amidst the world of tempting treats and guilty pleasures, one ingredient reigns supreme as the ultimate seductress: sugar. With its tantalizing sweetness and captivating allure, sugar weaves itself into the very fabric of our love affair with junk food. In this chapter, we delve into the intricate relationship between sugar and our indulgence in junk food, exploring the science, psychology, and cultural impact of this alluring ingredient.

The Sweet Symphony

From the first taste of a sugary delight, our taste buds are treated to a symphony of pleasure. Sugar triggers an immediate sensory response that transcends cultural boundaries and individual preferences. Its ability to activate our brain's reward centers creates a potent sensation of pleasure, akin to a cascade of euphoria that keeps us craving more.

The science behind this phenomenon lies in the brain's response to sugar. Consuming sugar releases dopamine – the neurotransmitter associated with pleasure and reward – creating a feedback loop that drives us to seek out more of this pleasurable sensation. As a result, we become entranced by the sweetness, locked in a cycle of desire and consumption.

The Art of Temptation: Sugar's Role in Craving

Sugar's seductive power goes beyond mere taste; it taps into the very mechanisms that drive our cravings. The more sugar we consume, the more our taste buds become acclimated to its sweetness. This phenomenon, known as sensory adaptation, leads us to seek out even sweeter and more intense flavors to achieve the same level of pleasure.

Moreover, sugar's impact on our blood sugar levels triggers a roller coaster of cravings. The rapid spike and subsequent crash in blood sugar levels create a cycle of hunger and desire, leading us to seek out quick sources of energy – often in the form of sugary snacks. This constant cycle perpetuates our cravings and keeps us trapped in the alluring embrace of junk food.

The Emotional Sweet Tooth

Sugar's role in our love affair with junk food extends beyond the realm of taste and physiology; it also plays a pivotal role in our emotional well-being. The consumption of sugary treats can provide a fleeting sense of comfort, a momentary reprieve from stress or sadness. In these moments, sugar becomes a source of emotional solace, offering a taste of pleasure that distracts us from our troubles.

The emotional connection to sugar is further magnified by cultural rituals and traditions. From birthday cakes to holiday sweets, sugar-laden treats often accompany moments of celebration and joy. These associations become imprinted in our memories, intertwining sugar with feelings of happiness and togetherness. As a result, sugar becomes more than a flavor; it becomes a conduit for the complex tapestry of human emotions.

Marketing Magic: Sugar's Role in Food Industry

The allure of sugar is also perpetuated by the food industry's strategic use of marketing and branding. The omnipresence of sugary products on supermarket shelves and the captivating imagery in advertisements contribute to our perception of sugar-laden treats as desirable and even necessary. Clever packaging, vibrant colors, and persuasive messaging create an aura of temptation that is hard to resist.

Furthermore, the deliberate manipulation of portion sizes and serving suggestions can amplify our consumption of sugar. Products are often designed to be easily consumed in one sitting, encouraging overindulgence and reinforcing the association between pleasure and excess. As a result, our relationship with sugar becomes intertwined with notions of abundance and fulfillment.

The Bittersweet Truth: Health Impact

While sugar's seductive allure is undeniable, it is accompanied by a bittersweet truth: its potential impact on our health. Excessive sugar consumption has been linked to a range of health issues, including obesity, type 2 diabetes, cardiovascular disease, and tooth decay. The addictive nature of sugar can lead to overconsumption, further exacerbating these health risks.

The rise of ultra-processed foods, which often contain hidden sugars, has led to a surge in our daily sugar intake. These foods are designed to be hyper-palatable, creating a perfect storm of cravings and consumption. As we continue to indulge in these sugary delights, the line between pleasure and potential harm becomes increasingly blurred.

Conclusion

Sugar's role in our love affair with junk food is a complex dance between pleasure and peril, desire and danger. It is a seductress that lures us with sweetness, ignites our senses, and captivates our emotions. From the moment it touches our taste buds to its impact on our health, sugar shapes our relationship with junk food in profound ways.

In the chapters that follow, we will delve deeper into the science of sugar addiction, explore strategies to navigate its allure, and uncover the surprising ways in which sugar impacts our well-being. As we continue our journey through the intricate world of junk food, we will gain insight into the mechanisms that drive our cravings and the steps we can take to cultivate a healthier relationship with this seductive ingredient. So, dear reader, join us as we peel back the layers of sweetness and explore the bittersweet truth behind sugar's role in our love affair with junk.

6.
FAST FOOD FRENZY: A HISTORICAL DIVE INTO DRIVE-THRUS AND MASCOTS

In the hustle and bustle of modern life, where time is a precious commodity and convenience is king, fast food has emerged as a cultural phenomenon that has transformed the way we eat and interact with food. The drive-thrus, iconic logos, and lovable mascots of fast food establishments have become integral parts of our culinary landscape. In this chapter, we embark on a historical journey through the evolution of fast food, exploring the origins of drive-thrus, the creation of beloved mascots, and the ways in which these elements have shaped our love affair with junk food.

The Birth of Speed: Origins of Drive-Thrus

The birth of the drive-thru, that iconic feature of the fast food industry, can be traced back to the mid-20th century. As post-World War II America embraced the automobile culture and families hit the road for leisure and adventure, a need arose for quick and convenient dining options. The drive-thru was a response to this demand, providing a way for busy travelers to grab a meal without leaving the comfort of their vehicles.

The first drive-thru restaurant, Red's Giant Hamburg in Missouri, opened its window in 1947. It was a modest establishment, offering hamburgers, cold drinks, and a streamlined service that catered to motorists on the go. This novel concept soon caught on, and other fast food chains followed suit, embracing the drive-thru as a central element of their business model.

The Mascot Magic: A World of Characters

Mascots have played a pivotal role in the fast food industry, captivating our imagination and becoming cultural touchstones that transcend their culinary origins. These characters are more than just advertising tools; they are icons that personify the essence of a brand and create a sense of familiarity and connection.

The birth of mascots can be attributed to a desire for differentiation and memorability in a competitive market. From the boisterous Colonel Sanders of KFC to the cheerful Ronald McDonald of McDonald's, these characters have become synonymous with their respective brands, evoking emotions ranging from joy and nostalgia to companionship and trust. They have the power to make us smile, to tug at our heartstrings, and even to shape our dining decisions.

Ronald McDonald and the Golden Arches: A Loveable Ambassador

No discussion of fast food mascots is complete without mentioning Ronald McDonald. Introduced in 1963 as a character to engage with children and families, Ronald McDonald quickly became the face of McDonald's and an enduring symbol of the brand's commitment to community and fun. With his vibrant red hair, yellow jumpsuit, and friendly demeanor, Ronald embodied the essence of childhood joy and adventure.

Ronald McDonald House Charities, established in 1974, further solidified the character's role as a positive force in the lives of families. The charity provides support to families of seriously ill children, reflecting McDonald's commitment to social responsibility and community involvement. The combination of entertainment, philanthropy, and familiarity has made Ronald McDonald a beloved and enduring figure in the fast food world.

Burger Kings and the King of Creepiness

Not all mascots take the path of joyful innocence. The Burger King mascot, often referred to as "The King," represents a departure from the typical cheerfulness associated with fast food characters. Introduced in the late 1950s, The King has undergone various iterations, from a jovial monarch to a more cryptic and enigmatic figure.

The King's campaigns have played with surrealism and offbeat humor, often straddling the line between amusing and unsettling. This departure from convention highlights the diverse ways in which mascots can capture our attention and leave a lasting impression, even if that impression veers toward the unconventional.

Wendy's and the Spokeswoman with Sass

Wendy's took a different approach by introducing a real-life persona as its brand spokesperson. Dave Thomas, the founder of Wendy's, became the face of the company in the late 1980s. His folksy charm, genuine demeanor, and personal anecdotes resonated with audiences, creating a connection that extended beyond the fast food counter.

Following Dave Thomas's passing, Wendy's continued its tradition of engaging spokespeople, notably with the introduction of the "Where's the Beef?" campaign in the 1980s. These spokespeople embodied the brand's witty and irreverent spirit, inviting consumers to engage in playful banter and sparking conversations that extended far beyond the realm of food.

The Global Impact of Icons

Fast food mascots and branding have transcended national borders, becoming symbols recognized and embraced around the world. These characters, through their universal appeal, have helped fast food chains establish a global presence and navigate cultural nuances.

However, this globalization has also sparked debates about cultural imperialism and the impact of Western food culture on local traditions. The introduction of American fast food mascots in international markets can symbolize more than just a meal; it can represent a collision of cultures, values, and culinary identities.

Conclusion

The history of fast food is a tale of innovation, convenience, and branding that has forever changed the way we approach dining. The introduction of drive-thrus, the creation of beloved mascots, and the global reach of these elements have woven themselves into the fabric of our culinary experience. These features, which often transcend the boundaries of food and advertising, have become cultural touchstones that reflect our love affair with junk food and the iconic symbols that define it.

In the chapters that follow, we will continue our exploration of the fast food frenzy, examining the psychology of cravings in the drive-thru line, uncovering the impact of convenience culture on our eating habits, and delving into the surprising ways in which fast food has shaped our society. As we peel back the layers of this culinary phenomenon, we will gain insight into the mechanisms that drive our indulgence and the ways in which fast food has become more than just a meal – it has become a symbol of our modern lifestyle and the complex desires that define it. So, dear reader, join us as we navigate the historical currents of the fast food industry and dive deeper into the world of drive-thrus, mascots, and the frenzy they inspire.

7.
PACKAGED TO PERFECTION: HOW MARKETING TRICKS US INTO CRAVING MORE

In the modern consumer landscape, where choices abound and attention spans are fleeting, the art of marketing has emerged as a powerful force that shapes our desires, influences our decisions, and even defines our cravings. The world of junk food is no exception, as advertisers employ a myriad of strategies to package their products to perfection, igniting our appetite for indulgence. In this chapter, we delve into the captivating world of food marketing, exploring the psychological techniques, design elements, and cultural cues that trick us into craving more of the very items we know we should resist.

The Illusion of Desirability

At the heart of food marketing lies the art of creating desire – the elusive quality that transforms ordinary products into objects of yearning. Through clever packaging, vibrant visuals, and strategic messaging, advertisers weave a narrative that speaks directly to our emotions, triggering a psychological response that heightens our perception of value and desirability.

Packaging, with its colors, textures, and typography, serves as the first point of contact between the consumer and the product. Bold, eye-catching designs and innovative packaging structures captivate our attention and evoke curiosity. These visual cues convey a sense of novelty and excitement, enticing us to explore further and consider the product as a potential indulgence.

The Science of Color and Imagery

Color psychology plays a pivotal role in food marketing, as different hues evoke specific emotions and associations. Warm, appetizing colors like red and orange stimulate feelings of hunger and excitement, while cool, soothing tones like blue may not be as effective in stimulating cravings. Advertisers harness these insights to create packaging that triggers a visceral response, making us more likely to reach for that enticing snack.

Imagery also plays a significant role in shaping our perceptions. The artful arrangement of ingredients, the glistening surface of a perfectly glazed pastry, or the rich, velvety texture of a chocolate bar – these images awaken our senses and engage our imagination. The brain's response to visual stimuli contributes to the allure of junk food, compelling us to indulge in the promise of sensory pleasure.

The Power of Branding

Branding is more than just a logo or a tagline; it's a comprehensive identity that shapes our relationship with a product. Brands become symbols of trust, familiarity, and consistency. The mere sight of a recognizable logo can trigger a flood of positive associations, tapping into our emotions and encouraging us to make a purchase.

Brand loyalty is cultivated through consistency in messaging and imagery. The repetition of a catchy jingle, the use of specific fonts, and the strategic placement of logos create a cohesive brand narrative that lodges itself in our memory. As a result, when we encounter a familiar brand on a store shelf, we feel an immediate sense of connection, making us more likely to choose that product over others.

Scarcity and FOMO

The psychology of scarcity and the fear of missing out (FOMO) are potent tools in the marketer's arsenal. Limited-time offers, seasonal releases, and exclusive promotions trigger our instinctive desire to obtain something rare or unique. The fear of missing out on a special treat or a unique flavor experience can create a sense of urgency, leading us to indulge in the moment rather than ponder the consequences.

This phenomenon is often amplified through social media, where images of friends enjoying a particular treat or discussing the latest food trend can trigger a sense of envy or curiosity. Advertisers capitalize on these emotions, using social media platforms to disseminate mouthwatering images and create a sense of community around their products.

The Subtle Art of Suggestion

Food marketing often involves subtle forms of suggestion that encourage us to make specific choices without explicitly telling us what to do. The positioning of products on store shelves, for instance, can influence our decisions. Eye-level placement of products, colorful displays, and enticing imagery can lead us to choose items that catch our attention, even if we hadn't initially planned to purchase them.

Similarly, the strategic placement of products near checkout counters or at the end of aisles is designed to capitalize on our impulse buying tendencies. These last-minute additions to our shopping carts are often prompted by the subconscious influence of our environment and the sensory cues that surround us.

Creating an Emotional Connection

Beyond the visual and sensory appeal, effective food marketing taps into our emotions, forging a deeper connection that extends beyond the product itself. Advertisers often create narratives that resonate with our aspirations, values, and personal experiences. Whether it's a heartwarming family meal, a celebration with friends, or a moment of personal indulgence, these narratives anchor the product in the context of our lives.

Furthermore, the use of relatable characters, heartwarming stories, or nostalgic elements can evoke a sense of familiarity and nostalgia. This emotional connection fosters a sense of trust and comfort, making us more likely to gravitate towards products that trigger positive emotions.

Conclusion

The world of food marketing is a landscape of visual artistry, psychological manipulation, and emotional connection that shapes our culinary desires and cravings. The packaging, branding, and messaging employed by advertisers play a pivotal role in creating a narrative that resonates with our senses and emotions, encouraging us to indulge in the allure of junk food.

In the chapters that follow, we will continue our exploration of the ways in which marketing influences our eating habits, delve into the science of food advertising, and uncover the surprising ways in which our perceptions of food are shaped by external cues. As we peel back the layers of packaging perfection, we will gain insight into the strategies that trick us into craving more and explore the power of mindfulness in navigating the world of culinary temptation. So, dear reader, join us as we dissect the art of food marketing and uncover the mechanisms that make us susceptible to its tantalizing influence.

8.

THE SCIENCE OF SALTY: WHY WE KEEP REACHING FOR THOSE CHIPS

The savory allure of salty snacks, from crispy potato chips to pretzels, holds a unique place in our love affair with junk food. The taste of salt triggers a symphony of sensations that captivate our taste buds and create an irresistible craving for more. In this chapter, we delve into the science behind our attraction to salty flavors, exploring the physiological, psychological, and cultural factors that contribute to our unending quest for that perfectly seasoned indulgence.

The Savoring Sensation: How Salt Tantalizes Our Tastes Buds

The allure of saltiness is deeply rooted in our evolutionary history. Salt is a fundamental nutrient essential for bodily functions such as nerve transmission, fluid balance, and muscle contractions. Our bodies are finely tuned to detect and crave salt, ensuring that we consume an adequate amount to maintain optimal health.

When salt makes contact with our taste buds, it triggers a complex sensory experience. The interaction between sodium ions and taste receptors stimulates neural pathways that send signals to the brain, creating a pleasurable sensation. This stimulation releases dopamine, the "feel-good" neurotransmitter, which fosters an immediate sense of reward and pleasure.

The Balance of Flavors: Umami and Salt

The allure of saltiness is often enhanced by its interaction with other taste sensations, particularly umami – the savory taste associated with foods rich in glutamate. Umami and saltiness share a synergistic relationship that amplifies the overall flavor experience. For example, a sprinkling of salt on a slice of tomato enhances its natural umami, creating a harmonious blend of flavors that captivates our palates.

The balanced interplay of sweet, salty, sour, bitter, and umami tastes creates a multidimensional experience that keeps our taste buds engaged and satisfied. This sensory symphony is the foundation of our attraction to salty foods, as our brains become conditioned to seek out these complex and rewarding flavor profiles.

The Pleasure Pathways: Salt and Brain Chemistry

The allure of saltiness is not confined to the realm of taste; it also delves into the intricate biochemistry of the brain. The consumption of salty foods triggers the release of opioids – natural chemicals that induce feelings of pleasure and euphoria. These opioids reinforce the reward pathways in the brain, creating a cycle of cravings and indulgence.

Furthermore, the brain's response to salt is intertwined with the regulation of appetite and satiety. Consuming salty foods can impact hormonal signaling that affects hunger and fullness, leading us to consume more than we might with other flavors. This intricate interplay of brain chemistry, taste perception, and physiological responses contributes to our relentless pursuit of the salty pleasures that junk food provides.

The Stealthy Salt Effect: Salt and Overconsumption

One of the challenges posed by saltiness is its ability to mask other flavors, making it easy to consume large quantities of food without noticing. The presence of salt can suppress bitter and sour tastes, making foods more palatable and encouraging overconsumption. This phenomenon, known as "flavor enhancement," can lead to mindless eating and contribute to the overconsumption of high-calorie, low-nutrient foods.

Moreover, the addictive nature of salt can lead to a phenomenon called "hedonic escalation." Over time, our taste buds become accustomed to higher levels of salt, causing us to seek out increasingly salty foods to achieve the same level of pleasure. This escalation can contribute to the overindulgence in salty snacks, perpetuating the cycle of cravings and consumption.

The Cultural and Psychological Impact

Salty flavors are deeply ingrained in many culinary traditions around the world. Salting, curing, and preserving foods have been fundamental practices for centuries, not only for flavor enhancement but also for food preservation. The cultural prevalence of salty foods has led to their integration into our eating habits and culinary preferences.

Beyond culture, saltiness also plays a role in emotional eating. Salty snacks are often associated with comfort and stress relief. The act of munching on chips or pretzels can provide a sense of solace and distraction, momentarily alleviating emotional discomfort. This emotional connection further solidifies the allure of salty junk food as a source of comfort in times of need.

The Salt Industry and Marketing Influence

The food industry's strategic use of salt in processed and packaged foods has contributed to our overconsumption of sodium. The salty taste can enhance the palatability of foods, mask undesirable flavors, and extend shelf life. As a result, salty snacks and processed foods become more appealing and convenient choices, especially when compared to whole, unprocessed options.

Marketing also plays a role in shaping our perceptions of saltiness. The "more is better" mentality can lead us to seek out foods with higher levels of salt, associating greater saltiness with enhanced flavor. This mindset can normalize excessive sodium consumption and contribute to our cravings for salty junk food.

Conclusion

The science of salty flavors is a complex interplay of sensory stimulation, brain chemistry, and cultural influences that contributes to our unending quest for indulgence. The allure of saltiness triggers a cascade of pleasurable sensations, reinforcing our cravings and driving us to seek out the irresistible flavors of junk food.

In the chapters that follow, we will continue our exploration of the science behind our cravings, delve into the impact of salt on our health, and uncover strategies to navigate the world of salty temptations. As we peel back the layers of our attraction to salty snacks, we will gain insight into the mechanisms that drive our desires and explore ways to cultivate a more mindful and balanced approach to our culinary indulgences. So, dear reader, join us as we uncover the secrets of the salty allure and embark on a journey to understand our complex relationship with junk food.

9.

FRANKENFOODS: DISSECTING THE BIZARRE INGREDIENTS LURKING IN OUR SNACKS

Amidst the world of vibrant packaging and mouthwatering flavors, a more sinister reality lurks within the realm of junk food: the presence of bizarre and often unpronounceable ingredients that make up the very fabric of these indulgent treats. From artificial colors to unrecognizable additives, the junk food industry has introduced a host of unconventional components that raise questions about their origins, safety, and impact on our health. In this chapter, we embark on a journey to dissect the world of "Frankenfoods," exploring the strange and sometimes unsettling ingredients that hide behind the enticing facade of our favorite snacks.

The Synthetic Symphony: Artificial Colors and Flavors

The allure of brightly colored candies, vibrant chips, and dazzling desserts often rests on the presence of artificial colors and flavors. These synthetic additives create a multisensory experience that engages our visual and gustatory senses, making junk food not only delicious but also visually captivating.

Artificial colors, often identified by numerical codes on ingredient labels, are used to mimic natural colors or enhance the visual appeal of food products. While they add an element of excitement to our snacks, concerns have been raised about their safety. Some artificial colors have been associated with hyperactivity in children and allergic reactions, prompting debates about their role in our culinary landscape.

Similarly, artificial flavors are designed to mimic natural taste sensations, often amplifying and enhancing the flavors of a product. The use of these synthetic flavors can mask the absence of real ingredients and create an addictive quality that keeps us reaching for more. However, the reliance on artificial flavors raises questions about the integrity and authenticity of the food we consume.

The Curious Case of Preservatives

Preservatives play a crucial role in extending the shelf life of processed foods and snacks, ensuring that they remain edible for extended periods. While this function may seem practical, the presence of certain preservatives has raised concerns about their potential health risks.

One group of preservatives, known as "BHA" and "BHT," is commonly used to prevent the oxidation of fats and oils in snacks. However, these additives have been linked to potential carcinogenic effects and adverse health outcomes. As we indulge in our favorite packaged treats, we may inadvertently be consuming ingredients that could have long-term implications for our well-being.

Navigating the Sea of Sweeteners

The pursuit of sweetness without the caloric consequences has given rise to an array of artificial sweeteners. These sugar substitutes promise the tantalizing taste of sweetness without the associated energy intake, making them attractive options for those seeking to manage their weight or control their blood sugar levels.

While artificial sweeteners offer a seemingly guilt-free way to enjoy sweet flavors, questions remain about their impact on our health. Some studies suggest that artificial sweeteners may influence our metabolism, appetite, and gut bacteria composition, potentially leading to unintended consequences. As we savor the sweetness of our favorite sugar-free treats, we find ourselves entangled in a complex web of potential health risks and benefits.

The Mystery of Texturizers and Emulsifiers

Texturizers and emulsifiers are lesser-known components that play a significant role in the composition of junk food. These additives are responsible for creating the desired texture, mouthfeel, and consistency of processed snacks, enhancing their appeal and palatability.

However, the use of texturizers and emulsifiers has raised concerns about their impact on our digestive health. Some emulsifiers, for instance, have been linked to disruptions in gut bacteria and inflammation. The hidden influence of these additives on our bodies highlights the intricate web of interactions that occur within the realm of processed and packaged foods.

Genetically Modified Organisms (GMOs): Unseen Alterations

The advent of genetically modified organisms (GMOs) has introduced a new layer of complexity to our food supply, with potentially far-reaching consequences. GMOs involve the manipulation of an organism's DNA to introduce desirable traits, such as resistance to pests or increased yield.

While GMOs have been praised for their potential to address global food security challenges, concerns linger about their long-term impact on human health and the environment. The presence of genetically modified ingredients in our snacks raises questions about transparency, labeling, and the potential risks associated with consuming these altered organisms.

Understanding Ingredient Lists: Navigating the Unknown

The ingredient list on food packaging can be a daunting landscape of unfamiliar terms and technical jargon. Deciphering these lists is crucial for making informed choices about the foods we consume. However, the complexity of ingredient names and the use of pseudonyms can make it challenging for consumers to truly understand what they are putting into their bodies.

In recent years, there has been a growing demand for transparency and clean labeling, prompting some food manufacturers to eliminate or reduce the use of artificial additives. This shift reflects consumers' desire for products that are made with recognizable and wholesome ingredients, emphasizing the importance of informed decision-making in our culinary choices.

Conclusion

The world of "Frankenfoods" is a realm of mystery and complexity, where unconventional ingredients hide beneath the surface of our favorite snacks. From artificial colors and flavors to preservatives, sweeteners, and texturizers, these additives play a significant role in shaping the taste, appearance, and appeal of junk food. As we peel back the layers of our indulgent treats, we uncover a tapestry of ingredients that raise questions about their origins, safety, and impact on our well-being.

In the chapters that follow, we will continue our exploration of the hidden elements that compose our favorite junk foods, delve into the science of food additives, and uncover strategies to navigate the world of processed and packaged snacks. As we gain insight into the complexity of ingredient lists and their potential implications, we will embark on a journey to cultivate a more conscious and informed approach to our culinary choices. So, dear reader, join us as we dissect the world of "Frankenfoods" and explore the mechanisms that drive our cravings and shape our relationship with junk food.

10.
HEALTH HALO HOAX: WHEN "ORGANIC" AND "NATURAL" DON'T MEAN HEALTHY

In a world where health-consciousness and nutritional awareness are on the rise, food labels adorned with terms like "organic," "natural," and "whole" can create a perception of virtuousness and healthfulness. However, the reality behind these labels is often more complex, and the allure of the "health halo" can lead us down a deceptive path. In this chapter, we unveil the truth behind the health halo phenomenon, exploring how terms like "organic" and "natural" can mislead us, the factors contributing to this deceptive marketing, and the ways in which our perceptions of health are shaped by these labels.

The Temptation of the Health Halo

The concept of the health halo revolves around the idea that certain labels create a positive perception of a product's healthfulness, leading consumers to make choices based on these perceptions rather than a comprehensive understanding of nutritional value. Labels such as "organic" and "natural" have the power to bestow an aura of wholesomeness and virtuousness upon products, regardless of their actual nutritional content.

This phenomenon can lead us to overconsume products under the illusion that they are healthier than they truly are. A bag of organic potato chips, for instance, might still be high in unhealthy fats and sodium, but the "organic" label can create a perception that these chips are a healthier alternative to conventional ones.

Decoding Organic: More Than Just Pesticide-Free

The term "organic" is often associated with healthier and more environmentally friendly options. Organic foods are grown without synthetic pesticides, herbicides, and genetically modified organisms (GMOs), and they adhere to strict guidelines set by certifying bodies. While organic farming practices can have environmental benefits and reduce exposure to certain chemicals, it's important to recognize that "organic" doesn't necessarily equate to a healthier or more nutritious product.

The health halo surrounding organic labels can lead to a false sense of security, causing us to overlook other important factors such as calorie content, sugar levels, and overall nutritional value. The perception that organic automatically means healthy can divert our attention from making well-informed dietary choices.

The Allure of "Natural" and "Clean" Labels

The term "natural" is another label that can evoke feelings of healthfulness and purity. Many consumers associate "natural" with whole, minimally processed ingredients. However, the FDA's definition of "natural" is vague and open to interpretation, allowing food manufacturers to use the label even for products that contain additives, preservatives, and artificial ingredients.

Similarly, the term "clean" has gained traction as a label associated with products that are free from artificial additives and chemicals. While the intention behind the "clean" label is to promote transparency and simplicity, it can also contribute to the health halo phenomenon. Consumers may interpret "clean" as a marker of superior nutritional quality, overlooking other critical aspects of a product's composition.

Portion Distortion and Health Halo

The health halo can also influence our perception of portion sizes. When a food is labeled as "organic," "natural," or "healthy," we may be more likely to consume larger portions under the assumption that these foods are inherently better for us. This phenomenon, known as portion distortion, can lead to overconsumption of calories, sugars, and unhealthy fats, ultimately undermining our efforts to make nutritious choices.

The health halo can also extend to restaurants and dining out. Dishes labeled as "light," "low-fat," or "natural" may lead us to underestimate their calorie content and overlook potential hidden sources of sugar and sodium. As a result, our perception of healthiness can be skewed, leading us to make dietary choices that don't align with our nutritional goals.

The Influence of Marketing and Packaging

The health halo phenomenon is often perpetuated by savvy marketing and packaging strategies. Advertisers leverage terms like "organic," "natural," and "clean" to create an emotional connection with consumers and position products as superior choices. The use of earthy colors, rustic imagery, and evocative language can further enhance the perception of healthfulness.

Furthermore, packaging designs that emphasize natural elements, such as images of farm fields or fresh produce, can create an association between the product and a wholesome lifestyle. These visual cues tap into our desire to make choices that align with our values, making us more susceptible to the allure of the health halo.

Consumer Empowerment: Reading Beyond the Labels

Navigating the world of food labels requires a critical and discerning eye. While labels like "organic" and "natural" can provide valuable information, they should not be the sole criteria for determining a product's healthfulness. Reading beyond the labels involves considering factors such as portion sizes, ingredient lists, and overall nutritional content.

Educating ourselves about the various terms used in food labeling is essential for making informed choices. Understanding the nuances of terms like "organic," "natural," "clean," and others empowers us to make decisions that align with our health and nutritional goals. Additionally, becoming familiar with ingredients and their potential health implications allows us to evaluate products based on their true nutritional value.

Conclusion

The health halo phenomenon is a testament to the power of marketing and labeling in shaping our perceptions of food. Labels like "organic" and "natural" evoke feelings of healthfulness and virtue, often leading us to make choices based on these perceptions rather than a comprehensive understanding of nutritional content. The allure of the health halo can divert our attention from other critical factors, such as portion sizes, calorie content, and overall composition.

In the chapters that follow, we will continue our exploration of the complexities of food labeling, delve into the psychology of healthy eating, and uncover strategies to navigate the world of deceptive marketing. As we peel back the layers of the health halo, we will gain insight into the mechanisms that influence our perceptions of health and explore ways to cultivate a more mindful and informed approach to our dietary choices. So, dear reader, join us as we debunk the myths of health labels and embark on a journey to uncover the truth behind the deceptive allure

of "organic" and "natural" in the world of junk
food.

11.
A GLOBAL GLUTTONY: EXPLORING JUNK FOOD'S WORLDWIDE IMPACT

Junk food's appeal knows no boundaries. From the bustling streets of urban metropolises to the tranquil villages of remote corners of the world, the allure of indulgent treats transcends cultures, languages, and borders. In this chapter, we embark on a journey to explore the global impact of junk food, examining how its proliferation has transformed societies, shaped dietary habits, and contributed to a complex web of health, social, and environmental challenges.

The Fast Food Diaspora: A Global Culinary Landscape

The rise of global fast food chains has reshaped the culinary landscape of countries far and wide. The introduction of familiar brands and flavors has created a sense of familiarity in foreign settings, offering a taste of the Western lifestyle and convenience culture. The ubiquity of McDonald's arches, KFC's buckets, and Pizza Hut's delivery boxes is a testament to the global appeal of fast food.

While fast food chains often tailor their menus to local tastes, the spread of these establishments can come at a cost. Traditional dietary patterns and local ingredients may take a back seat to the convenience and familiarity of fast food. This shift can contribute to the displacement of traditional foods, potentially affecting cultural identity and culinary heritage.

The Globalization of Taste: A Two-Way Street

The influence of global fast food is not a one-sided affair. As junk food spreads its influence, local cuisines also impact the world of fast food. Fast food menus in different countries often incorporate regional flavors and ingredients to cater to local tastes. This mutual exchange has led to the creation of unique fusion dishes that blend traditional elements with fast food convenience.

However, the globalization of taste also raises concerns about the homogenization of dietary habits. The prominence of junk food in various parts of the world can contribute to a loss of dietary diversity, potentially leading to health issues and undermining the unique nutritional benefits that diverse cuisines provide.

Health and Social Consequences

The global consumption of junk food has far-reaching health implications. The proliferation of high-calorie, low-nutrient foods has contributed to rising rates of obesity, diabetes, and other diet-related diseases on a global scale. The ease of access to these foods, coupled with aggressive marketing strategies, has created a perfect storm that fosters overconsumption and poor nutritional choices.

Furthermore, the social consequences of junk food's impact are equally significant. Health disparities often emerge as low-income communities are disproportionately affected by the accessibility and affordability of unhealthy foods. This phenomenon perpetuates a cycle of poor health outcomes and economic challenges, further exacerbating existing inequalities.

Environmental Impact and Sustainability

Junk food's worldwide reach also takes a toll on the environment. The production, transportation, and packaging of processed and packaged foods contribute to greenhouse gas emissions, resource depletion, and waste generation. The global demand for ingredients like palm oil, which is commonly used in snack foods, has led to deforestation and habitat destruction in some regions.

Additionally, the reliance on animal agriculture for meat-based junk food options contributes to the environmental strain of livestock production. The global appetite for beef, chicken, and other meat products has implications for land use, water consumption, and deforestation, amplifying the environmental challenges associated with junk food consumption.

Cultural Identity and Identity Loss

As junk food infiltrates local markets and diets, it can also impact cultural identity and traditional food practices. The prominence of global fast food chains can overshadow local culinary traditions, leading to a loss of cultural authenticity and eroding the unique flavors and techniques that define a region's cuisine.

Furthermore, the homogenization of dietary habits can lead to a loss of individual identity as traditional foods and flavors are replaced by mass-produced and standardized options. This phenomenon raises questions about the preservation of cultural heritage and the ways in which globalization shapes personal and collective identities.

Education and Empowerment: Navigating the Global Junk Food Landscape

Addressing the global impact of junk food requires a multifaceted approach that encompasses education, policy change, and individual empowerment. Public health campaigns, nutritional education, and efforts to promote local and sustainable food systems are crucial components of this strategy.

Policy interventions, such as taxes on unhealthy foods and restrictions on marketing to children, can help create an environment that encourages healthier dietary choices. These measures can also address the disparities in access to nutritious foods, particularly in underserved communities.

Empowering individuals to make informed choices in the face of global junk food influence is essential. Building food literacy, teaching critical thinking about marketing tactics, and promoting culinary skills can enable people to navigate the complex landscape of dietary options and prioritize their health and well-being.

Conclusion

The global impact of junk food is a complex tapestry of cultural exchange, dietary shifts, health challenges, and environmental consequences. The proliferation of processed and packaged foods, alongside the influence of global fast food chains, has transformed societies, reshaped culinary traditions, and contributed to a range of health and social issues.

In the chapters that follow, we will continue our exploration of the global impact of junk food, delving into the role of government policies, international efforts, and personal choices in addressing these challenges. As we peel back the layers of junk food's worldwide influence, we will gain insight into the mechanisms that drive its consumption, explore potential solutions, and embark on a journey to cultivate a more conscious and responsible approach to our dietary habits. So, dear reader, join us as we unravel the global gluttony of junk food and explore the ways in which it shapes our world – from local tables to international markets.

12.

NAVIGATING THE DRIVE-THRU: A HUMOROUS GUIDE TO FAST FOOD LINGO

Ah, the drive-thru – that magical window where hunger meets convenience, and where our taste buds embark on a journey through the land of burgers, fries, and milkshakes. But let's face it, ordering at the drive-thru can sometimes feel like trying to decipher a secret code. From quirky lingo to curious abbreviations, the fast food world has its own language, and navigating it can be an adventure in itself. In this chapter, we embark on a humorous exploration of the fast food lexicon, decoding the quirky phrases and playful terms that make up the drive-thru dialogue.

The Lingo Lexicon: A Crash Course in Fast Food Speak

Before we dive into the specifics, let's establish some basics. The drive-thru lexicon is a mishmash of terms, abbreviations, and slang that may leave you feeling like you've stumbled into a linguistic amusement park. But don't worry – we're here to guide you through the twists and turns of this linguistic rollercoaster.

1. The Combo Conundrum: Fast food joints love their combos, and for good reason – they're a one-stop solution for a complete meal. But deciphering the combo codes can feel like cracking a safe. You've got your small #1, medium #3, large #5, and let's not even talk about the "upsize" option. Just remember, the number refers to the meal, the size refers to the fries and drink, and the experience is all about embracing the chaos.

2. Hold the Pickles, Please: Customization is king in the drive-thru universe. If you're particular about your toppings, just throw in a "hold the" before the ingredient you'd rather skip. Whether it's pickles, onions, or the entire garden, this simple phrase grants you the power to curate your culinary masterpiece.

3. The Fry Game: Fries – the crunchy, salty accomplices to your main course. But the fry game can get tricky. Do you want them regular, curly, or waffle? And what about sizes – small, medium, or large? Just remember, there's no wrong choice in the fry department. They're all winners in the end.

4. The Special Request Shuffle: Got a special request? Fear not. Fast food employees are the masters of improvisation. Whether it's a patty swap, a sauce switcheroo, or the mythical "secret menu" item you heard about online, don't be afraid to unleash your inner food artist. Your drive-thru experience is your canvas.

Flipping the Script: A Peek Behind the Counter

Now that we've covered the basics, let's flip the script and take a peek behind the counter. Fast food workers are the unsung heroes of the drive-thru world, juggling orders, assembling meals, and maintaining their cool in the face of hangry customers. Their lingo is a dance of efficiency and camaraderie, and it's a delightful glimpse into the inner workings of the fast food universe.

1. The "Bun Buzzer": Ever wondered how your burger arrives fresh and warm? That's the magic of the "bun buzzer." When an order is placed, the kitchen team coordinates with the front counter, ensuring that your buns (and other ingredients) are perfectly timed for assembly. It's a symphony of teamwork and timing, all for your gustatory delight.

2. The "Ticket Tango": Behind the counter, the order screen is a dance floor of digital tickets, each representing a customer's culinary desires. The "ticket tango" is the art of interpreting these digital symphonies, translating them into delicious reality, and sending them on their way to the eagerly awaiting drive-thru window.

3. The "Sauce Samba": Sauces are the spice of life, and fast food workers have mastered the art of the "sauce samba." From ketchup to mayo, special sauces to spicy delights, they navigate an array of condiments with grace and precision, ensuring that every order is sauced to perfection.

4. The "Fry Fandango": Fries are the pièce de résistance of many fast food meals, and the "fry fandango" is a dance of portioning, frying, and salting that results in those golden, crispy delights that have won the hearts of fry enthusiasts around the world.

Putting the "Fun" in Fast Food Lingo

Now that we've taken a whirlwind tour through the fast food lingo landscape, it's time to put the "fun" in fast food lingo. Embracing the quirkiness and playfulness of the drive-thru dialogue can turn your dining experience into a delightful adventure.

1. The Decoder Ring: If you're feeling particularly adventurous, why not create your own fast food decoder ring? Craft a list of your favorite fast food terms, complete with translations and your own humorous interpretations. It's a surefire way to inject some chuckles into your drive-thru escapades.

2. The Accidental Order: Ever tried the "accidental order" game? Simply close your eyes, point at the menu, and order whatever

your finger lands on. Who knows, you might discover a new favorite or unleash your inner culinary explorer.

3. **The Playful Pronunciations**: Don't be afraid to have a little fun with your pronunciation. Order that "double-double cheesy extravaganza" or the "mega-munchy munch-o-rama." It's a guaranteed way to bring a smile to both your face and the drive-thru attendant's.

4. **The Impromptu Rap**: Feeling musical? Why not turn your order into an impromptu rap or song? Let your inner lyricist loose and serenade the drive-thru with your lyrical masterpiece. Bonus points for rhyming "extra cheese" with "please"!

Conclusion

Navigating the drive-thru is not just about getting your hands on a delicious meal – it's an opportunity for a linguistic adventure, a chance to embrace the playful and quirky lingo that defines the fast food world. So the next time you roll up to the drive-thru window, let your inner foodie poet shine, and remember, whether you're craving a "cheesy delight" or a "crunchy munch-a-thon," the fast food lingo is your ticket to a humorous and memorable dining experience. Bon appétit, dear reader, and may your drive-thru adventures be filled with laughter and delight!

13.
BREAKING FREE: OVERCOMING THE CLUTCHES OF JUNK FOOD ADDICTION

Picture this: you're lounging on the couch, Netflix on, a bag of chips in one hand and a sugary soda in the other. Sound familiar? Junk food addiction is a reality many of us face, and breaking free from its clutches can feel like attempting to escape quicksand. But fear not, for in this chapter, we embark on a journey of empowerment and transformation. We'll explore the science behind junk food addiction, understand the psychological factors that keep us hooked, and discover actionable strategies to break the cycle and reclaim control over our cravings.

The Science of Cravings: Unraveling the Addiction

Junk food addiction is not just a matter of willpower; it's deeply rooted in the brain's reward system. The rapid release of dopamine, the "feel-good" neurotransmitter, in response to sugar, salt, and unhealthy fats creates a cycle of pleasure and craving. Over time, our brains become wired to seek out these pleasurable sensations, leading to a cycle of dependence similar to that seen in substance addiction.

This physiological response is further exacerbated by the food industry's strategic use of flavor enhancers, additives, and high levels of salt and sugar. The combination of sensory stimulation and biochemical reactions creates a perfect storm of addiction, making it increasingly challenging to resist the allure of junk food.

The Psychology of Temptation: Triggers and Craving Loops

Understanding the psychological triggers that lead to junk food consumption is a key step in breaking free from addiction. Stress, emotions, boredom, and even environmental cues can all activate the brain's reward system, triggering cravings and a desire for instant gratification.

Craving loops are another psychological phenomenon that reinforces junk food addiction. The act of giving in to a craving provides temporary relief, followed by feelings of guilt and regret. This emotional rollercoaster can lead to an endless cycle of cravings, consumption, and guilt, creating a vicious loop that perpetuates the addiction.

Strategies for Breaking the Cycle

Breaking free from junk food addiction requires a multifaceted approach that addresses both the physiological and psychological aspects of cravings. Here are some strategies to help you reclaim control and overcome the clutches of addiction:

1. Mindful Awareness: Start by becoming mindful of your cravings and triggers. Keep a journal to track your emotions, situations, and thoughts when cravings strike. Identifying patterns can help you anticipate and manage triggers more effectively.

2. **Rewire Your Brain:** Just as the brain can be wired for addiction, it can also be rewired for healthier habits. Gradually reduce your intake of junk food while incorporating whole, nutrient-rich foods. Over time, your brain will begin to associate healthier options with pleasure and satisfaction.

3. **Break the Cycle:** When a craving hits, engage in an activity that disrupts the craving loop. Go for a walk, meditate, or practice deep breathing. These activities can help divert your attention away from the craving and give your brain a chance to reset.

4. **Opt for Substitutes:** Replace unhealthy snacks with nutritious alternatives. Keep a variety of fruits, vegetables, nuts, and whole grains on hand to satisfy your cravings in a healthier way.

5. **Practice Delay:** When a craving strikes, commit to delaying your response for a set period of time, such as 10 minutes. Use this time to evaluate the craving and decide if it's truly worth indulging.

6. **Seek Support:** Enlist the support of friends, family, or a support group. Sharing your journey with others can provide accountability, encouragement, and a sense of community.

7. **Professional Guidance:** If you find that your addiction is deeply entrenched and difficult to overcome on your own, consider seeking the guidance of a healthcare professional or therapist. They can provide tailored strategies and support to help you break free from the cycle of addiction.

The Path to Freedom: Embracing a New Relationship with Food

Breaking free from junk food addiction is not just about eliminating unhealthy snacks; it's about cultivating a new relationship with food and nourishing your body in a way that promotes well-being. This journey is one of self-discovery, self-compassion, and empowerment.

1. **Mindful Eating:** Practice mindful eating by savoring each bite, paying attention to flavors, textures, and sensations. Eating

slowly and tuning into your body's hunger and fullness cues can help you make conscious choices and prevent overindulgence.

2. Balanced Nutrition: Focus on a balanced and varied diet that includes a variety of nutrient-rich foods. Incorporate whole grains, lean proteins, fruits, vegetables, and healthy fats to provide your body with the essential nutrients it needs.

3. Culinary Exploration: Embrace the joy of cooking and experimenting with new recipes. Engaging in the process of meal preparation can deepen your connection to the food you consume and foster a sense of empowerment.

4. Self-Compassion: Be kind to yourself throughout the journey. Overcoming addiction is a process, and setbacks are a natural part of the process. Instead of dwelling on slip-ups, focus on your progress and celebrate your successes.

5. Long-Term Sustainability: Remember that breaking free from junk food addiction is not a

temporary endeavor; it's a lifelong commitment to your health and well-being. Strive for long-term sustainability by adopting habits that you can maintain over time.

Conclusion

Breaking free from the clutches of junk food addiction is a transformative journey that requires dedication, self-awareness, and a willingness to embrace change. By understanding the science behind cravings, addressing psychological triggers, and implementing practical strategies, you can regain control over your relationship with food and experience the empowerment of making conscious choices.

In the chapters that follow, we will continue our exploration of the complex world of junk food addiction, delve into the role of societal factors and marketing influence, and uncover strategies to create a sustainable and balanced approach to eating. As we peel back the layers of addiction and empowerment, we will gain insight into the mechanisms that drive our cravings and embark on a journey to reclaim our health, well-being, and sense of agency. So, dear reader, join us as we break free from the clutches of junk food addiction and embrace a new path toward a healthier and more fulfilling life.

14.

THE EMOTIONAL EATING ROLLER COASTER: FROM COMFORT TO REGRET

Have you ever found solace in a pint of ice cream after a tough day, or sought refuge in a bag of chips when stress comes knocking? Emotional eating is a journey through complex emotions, a roller coaster that takes us from comfort to regret. In this chapter, we delve into the intricate world of emotional eating, exploring the psychological triggers that drive us to seek comfort in food, the impact of this behavior on our well-being, and strategies to break free from its grip.

Emotional Eating Unveiled: The Comfort Seeker Within

Emotional eating is a coping mechanism rooted in the desire for comfort and relief from emotional distress. It involves turning to food as a source of solace, often triggered by stress, sadness, boredom, or even happiness. The act of eating provides a temporary escape from negative emotions, offering a fleeting sense of control and pleasure.

The connection between emotions and food is deeply ingrained, often dating back to our earliest experiences. Comforting foods, whether a warm bowl of soup or a favorite childhood treat, can evoke feelings of safety and security. Over time, this association between food and comfort becomes a go-to response when emotions run high.

The Emotional Eating Cycle: From Triggers to Guilt

Emotional eating is a cycle with distinct phases, each contributing to the roller coaster journey:

1. **Trigger:** Emotional eating begins with an emotional trigger – stress, anxiety, loneliness, or even joy. These emotions create a sense of discomfort or unease, prompting the urge to seek relief.

2. Craving: The emotional trigger activates cravings for specific comfort foods. These foods are often high in sugar, fat, and salt – ingredients that trigger the brain's reward system and offer a sense of instant gratification.

3. Consumption: Succumbing to the craving, we consume the comfort food. The act of eating provides a momentary distraction from the underlying emotions and offers a sense of temporary relief.

4. Guilt and Regret: After indulging, feelings of guilt and regret often follow. The initial comfort is replaced by negative emotions, creating a cycle of guilt that can perpetuate the pattern of emotional eating.

The Emotional Eating Spectrum: Beyond Negative Emotions

While emotional eating is commonly associated with negative emotions, it can also be triggered by positive feelings. Celebratory events, social gatherings, and even moments of happiness can prompt overconsumption of unhealthy foods. This spectrum of emotional triggers highlights the complexity of our relationship with food and the myriad ways in which emotions influence our eating behaviors.

Breaking Free from Emotional Eating: Strategies for Resilience

Breaking the cycle of emotional eating requires a multifaceted approach that addresses the underlying emotions, develops healthier coping mechanisms, and cultivates self-awareness. Here are strategies to help you navigate the emotional eating roller coaster and regain control over your relationship with food:

1. Mindful Awareness: Begin by cultivating mindfulness around your eating habits and emotions. When a craving arises, take a moment to pause and reflect on the emotions driving the urge to eat. Developing this awareness can help you differentiate between physical hunger and emotional hunger.

2. Emotional Regulation: Instead of turning to food as a primary coping mechanism, explore

alternative ways to regulate your emotions. Engage in activities such as journaling, deep breathing, meditation, or physical exercise to manage stress and anxiety.

3. Healthy Coping Mechanisms: Create a toolkit of healthy coping mechanisms that provide comfort without resorting to food. Engage in hobbies, connect with loved ones, practice relaxation techniques, or engage in creative outlets that offer a sense of fulfillment.

4. Nutrient-Rich Choices: Opt for nutrient-rich foods that nourish your body and support emotional well-being. Incorporate fruits, vegetables, whole grains, and lean proteins into your meals to provide sustained energy and stabilize mood.

5. Self-Compassion: Be gentle with yourself on this journey. Recognize that emotional eating is a common response to emotional distress and that breaking the cycle takes time. Instead of berating yourself for slip-ups, practice self-compassion and focus on progress.

6. Seek Support: If emotional eating feels overwhelming, consider seeking support from a therapist or counselor. Professional guidance can provide tailored strategies to address underlying emotional triggers and develop healthier coping mechanisms.

Reclaiming Emotional Resilience: A Journey of Empowerment

Breaking free from the emotional eating roller coaster is not just about curbing a behavior; it's a journey toward emotional resilience and self-empowerment. By understanding the triggers, developing healthier coping mechanisms, and fostering self-awareness, you can transform your relationship with food and regain control over your emotional responses.

In the chapters that follow, we will continue our exploration of the intricate landscape of emotional eating, delve into the role of societal influences and cultural factors, and uncover strategies to create a balanced and nourishing approach to eating. As we peel back the layers of emotional eating and empowerment, we will gain insight into the mechanisms that drive our cravings and embark on a journey to reclaim our emotional well-being and establish a harmonious connection with food. So, dear reader, join us as we navigate the emotional eating roller coaster and embrace a path toward emotional resilience and self-discovery.

15.

FORBIDDEN LOVE: TALES OF SNEAKING JUNK FOOD BEHIND HEALTH'S BACK

Imagine this clandestine scene: under the cloak of darkness, you tiptoe into the kitchen, hushed breaths punctuating the silence. Your heart races as you reach for that forbidden bag of chips, your fingers dancing over the crinkly packaging. You indulge in your secret vice, savoring every bite while glancing over your shoulder, as if health itself might catch you in the act. Welcome to the world of sneaking junk food behind health's back – a realm where pleasure and guilt collide. In this chapter, we unravel the tales of these covert indulgences, explore the psychology behind the forbidden love affair, and delve into strategies to navigate this delicate dance.

The Allure of Secrecy: The Forbidden Fruit

The allure of sneaking junk food is a fascinating interplay of pleasure and secrecy. The act of indulging in forbidden treats creates an adrenaline rush, a thrill akin to embarking on a secret adventure. The knowledge that you're deviating from your health goals adds an element of danger, heightening the experience.

This dynamic is reminiscent of a forbidden love affair, with the indulgence serving as the passionate rendezvous and the guilt as the emotional aftermath. The secrecy and excitement contribute to the appeal, but they also underscore the complex psychological underpinnings of this behavior.

The Psychology of Sneaking: Pleasure and Guilt

Sneaking junk food behind health's back is often driven by a tug-of-war between pleasure and guilt. The anticipation of the indulgence generates excitement and pleasure, while the act itself offers a brief escape from routine and restrictions. The taste of the forbidden is intensified by the backdrop of secrecy, creating a heightened sensory experience.

However, the aftermath is often colored by guilt and remorse. The momentary pleasure is quickly overshadowed by feelings of self-disgust and disappointment, leading to a cycle of emotional turmoil. This emotional rollercoaster mirrors the ebb and flow of a tumultuous relationship, where moments of bliss are followed by pangs of regret.

The Ritual of Sneaking: An Intricate Dance

Sneaking junk food is often accompanied by a ritualistic dance, complete with its own set of steps. From choosing the perfect hiding spot to orchestrating the timing of the indulgence, each element contributes to the clandestine nature of the act.

1. **The Covert Operation:** Planning the indulgence requires careful strategy. You time it just right – when no one's around, when you have the house to yourself, or perhaps in the dead of night. The secrecy adds an element of suspense, elevating the experience.

2. The Selection: Choosing the forbidden treat is a delicate decision. It's not just about what you're eating; it's about the thrill of breaking the rules. The act of selecting the indulgence is part of the anticipation, heightening the allure.

3. The Sensory Symphony: As you indulge, your senses are heightened. The flavors are intensified, and each bite becomes a sensory symphony. This heightened experience is a result of both the forbidden nature of the indulgence and the focus on the present moment.

4. The Aftermath: Once the indulgence is over, the emotional aftermath sets in. Guilt, regret, and a sense of betrayal accompany the pleasure. The emotional journey resembles the complexities of a romantic entanglement, complete with the push and pull of emotions.

Strategies for Navigating the Forbidden Love Affair

Breaking free from the cycle of sneaking junk food involves a nuanced approach that addresses both the psychological triggers and the emotional aftermath. Here are strategies to navigate this forbidden love affair and foster a healthier relationship with food:

1. Self-Reflection: Take time to reflect on the emotional and psychological factors driving your desire to sneak junk food. Are you using food as a coping mechanism? Are there underlying emotions you're trying to soothe? Identifying these triggers is a crucial step toward understanding your behavior.

2. Mindful Indulgence: Instead of sneaking, practice mindful indulgence. Choose a specific time and place to enjoy your treat, and savor every bite without guilt. Mindful eating allows you to experience pleasure without the emotional turmoil of secrecy.

3. Alternative Coping Mechanisms: Develop alternative coping mechanisms for dealing with stress, boredom, or emotions. Engage in activities such as exercise, journaling, or creative outlets to channel your emotions in a healthier way.

4. **Open Dialogue**: Consider opening up to a trusted friend, family member, or therapist about your struggles with sneaking junk food. Sharing your experiences can provide emotional support, accountability, and a sense of relief.

5. **Reevaluate Restrictions**: Reevaluate your approach to dietary restrictions. Strive for a balanced approach that allows for occasional indulgences without the need for secrecy. Denying yourself entirely can contribute to the allure of sneaking.

6. **Self-Compassion**: Practice self-compassion and forgiveness. Recognize that slipping into old habits is a natural part of the process. Instead of berating yourself, focus on learning from the experience and moving forward.

Transforming the Relationship: Empowerment and Freedom

Navigating the world of sneaking junk food behind health's back is a journey of transformation, one that involves unraveling the complexities of desire, guilt, and pleasure. By understanding the psychology behind this forbidden love affair, developing healthier coping mechanisms, and fostering self-awareness, you can reclaim control over your relationship with food.

In the chapters that follow, we will continue our exploration of the intricate landscape of dietary behaviors, delve into the impact of societal influences and cultural norms, and uncover strategies to create a harmonious and balanced approach to eating. As we peel back the layers of forbidden love and empowerment, we will gain insight into the mechanisms that shape our behaviors and embark on a journey to reclaim our sense of agency, freedom, and emotional well-being. So, dear reader, join us as we navigate the world of sneaking junk food behind health's back and embrace a path toward self-discovery and transformation.

16.
KITCHEN CONFESSIONS: DIY VERSIONS OF YOUR FAVORITE TRASHY TREATS

There's a certain allure to the world of trashy treats – those guilty pleasures that tantalize our taste buds with their sinful flavors and indulgent textures. But what if you could enjoy those beloved junk foods without the baggage of excess calories and questionable ingredients? Welcome to the realm of kitchen confessions, where we unlock the secrets to crafting your own DIY versions of trashy treats. In this chapter, we'll embark on a culinary adventure, exploring creative recipes that capture the essence of your favorite indulgences while embracing wholesome, nourishing ingredients.

Decoding the DIY Magic: Crafting Healthier Versions

The art of recreating trashy treats at home is a delightful blend of creativity, culinary ingenuity, and a touch of DIY magic. By deconstructing the flavors and textures that make these treats irresistible, you can create healthier versions that satisfy your cravings without compromising on taste.

The beauty of DIY versions lies in their adaptability. Whether you're seeking a crunchy, salty snack fix, a velvety dessert, or a savory comfort dish, the kitchen is your playground for experimentation. Armed with a bit of inspiration and a dash of culinary curiosity, you can embark on a journey of flavor discovery and redefine your relationship with these classic treats.

Trashy to Tasty: DIY Transformations

Let's dive into the world of kitchen confessions with a showcase of DIY versions of your favorite trashy treats:

1. Crunchy Cravings: Baked Veggie Chips

Bid adieu to store-bought potato chips and embark on a healthier snacking adventure with baked veggie chips. Thinly slice root vegetables like sweet potatoes, beets, or kale, season them with a sprinkle of olive oil and your favorite spices, and bake until crispy. These colorful chips offer a satisfying crunch while packing a nutritional punch.

2. Sweet Delights: Chia Seed Pudding Parfait

Indulge your sweet tooth with a chia seed pudding parfait that rivals the creaminess of traditional desserts. Mix chia seeds with your choice of milk, sweeten with a touch of honey or maple syrup, and let it thicken overnight. Layer the pudding with fresh fruits, granola, and a dollop of Greek yogurt for a guilt-free dessert that's both nourishing and delectable.

3. Comfort Classics: Cauliflower Mac and Cheese

Craving the creamy comfort of mac and cheese? Swap out pasta for cauliflower florets and create a cheesy sauce using a blend of nutritional yeast, low-fat milk, and a touch of mustard. The result? A velvety, savory dish that satisfies your comfort food cravings while incorporating a dose of veggie goodness.

4. Guilty Pleasure: Guilt-Free Ice Cream

Ice cream cravings met their match with guilt-free, homemade versions. Blend frozen bananas with a splash of almond milk and your favorite mix-ins – think berries, nuts, or dark chocolate chunks. The result is a luscious, creamy treat that offers the same indulgent satisfaction as traditional ice cream, minus the added sugars and artificial flavors.

The Joy of Culinary Exploration: Customizing Your Creations

What makes kitchen confessions truly remarkable is the joy of customization. These DIY versions provide a canvas for culinary creativity, allowing you to tailor each recipe to your taste preferences and dietary needs. Whether you're exploring plant-based options, reducing refined sugars, or incorporating nutrient-rich ingredients, the possibilities are as vast as your imagination.

1. **Flavor Fusion:** Experiment with a fusion of flavors by adding unexpected ingredients to your DIY treats. Infuse your baked veggie chips with a hint of smoked paprika or cumin, or elevate your chia seed pudding with a dash of cardamom or vanilla extract.

2. **Nutrient Boost:** Enhance the nutritional content of your creations by sneaking in nutrient-packed additions. Amp up the fiber in your cauliflower mac and cheese by tossing in some spinach or broccoli, or add a sprinkle of flaxseeds to your guilt-free ice cream for an omega-3 boost.

3. **Portion Control:** DIY versions also grant you the power of portion control. By crafting smaller servings of your favorite treats, you can savor the flavors without overindulging. This mindful approach allows you to enjoy the essence of the treat while maintaining a balanced approach to eating.

Embracing the Kitchen Confessions Lifestyle

Kitchen confessions extend beyond a collection of recipes; they embody a lifestyle that celebrates culinary exploration, mindful choices, and a harmonious relationship with food. By embracing the art of recreating trashy treats at home, you cultivate a sense of empowerment and agency over your dietary decisions.

1. Mindful Indulgence: Kitchen confessions encourage mindful indulgence, where you savor each bite and fully appreciate the flavors and textures of your creations. This mindful approach fosters a deeper connection to your food and promotes a sense of satisfaction.

2. Creativity and Joy: Engaging in DIY cooking allows you to tap into your creativity and experience the joy of culinary experimentation. As you craft your own versions of favorite treats, you'll find pleasure in the process of creation and a newfound appreciation for wholesome ingredients.

3. Sustainable Choices: Embracing kitchen confessions aligns with a sustainable approach to eating. By preparing your own treats, you reduce reliance on packaged and processed foods, contribute to waste

reduction, and make choices that promote both personal and planetary well-being.

Conclusion

Kitchen confessions offer a window into a world where indulgence meets nourishment, and creativity intersects with culinary exploration. By crafting your own DIY versions of trashy treats, you embark on a journey that redefines your relationship with food, empowers you to make mindful choices, and invites you to savor the pleasure of flavors and textures.

In the chapters that follow, we will continue our exploration of the dynamic realm of culinary creativity, delve into the impact of societal influences on our dietary behaviors, and uncover strategies to foster a balanced and wholesome approach to eating. As we peel back the layers of indulgence and empowerment, we will gain insight into the mechanisms that shape our culinary choices and embark on a journey to reclaim our sense of agency, joy, and well-being. So, dear reader, join us as we immerse ourselves in the art of kitchen confessions and embrace a path toward culinary fulfillment and self-discovery.

17.
WACKY CRAVINGS: THE STRANGEST JUNK FOOD COMBINATIONS WE CAN'T RESIST

Imagine a world where pickles cozy up to peanut butter, where chocolate finds an unexpected partner in hot sauce, and where potato chips make their way into ice cream sundaes. Welcome to the realm of wacky cravings – a world where culinary boundaries are pushed, and the most unconventional junk food combinations become irresistible delights. In this chapter, we embark on a journey to explore the quirkiest, most peculiar, and surprisingly satisfying junk food pairings that tickle our taste buds and challenge our culinary norms.

The Curious Allure of Wacky Cravings

Wacky cravings are a testament to the unpredictable and often delightful nature of our taste preferences. These unusual combinations defy logic and tradition, yet they captivate our senses and leave us craving more. The allure lies in the juxtaposition of flavors, textures, and aromas that create a symphony of sensations, leading to an unexpected harmony that defies expectations.

The phenomenon of wacky cravings is a testament to the human palate's versatility and openness to experimentation. It showcases our willingness to embrace the unorthodox and our curiosity to explore uncharted flavor territories. Whether born out of necessity or culinary curiosity, these combinations challenge our preconceived notions of what constitutes a satisfying indulgence.

The Psychology Behind the Mash-Up

The psychology behind wacky cravings is a fascinating exploration of how our brains interpret and respond to taste experiences. The human palate is a complex sensory organ that can discern a myriad of flavors, both complementary and contrasting. Wacky cravings often play on the principle of contrast, where unexpected pairings create a unique and memorable eating experience.

Additionally, the element of surprise plays a significant role in the appeal of wacky cravings. When we encounter a combination that defies our expectations, our curiosity is piqued, and we're drawn to explore further. The anticipation of an unconventional flavor profile adds an element of excitement and novelty to the eating experience, making it all the more enjoyable.

The Chronicles of Wacky Cravings: A Culinary Adventure

Let's embark on a culinary adventure and explore some of the most intriguing wacky junk food combinations that have captured our imaginations:

1. PB & P: Peanut Butter and Pickles

This unconventional pairing combines the creamy richness of peanut butter with the tangy crunch of pickles. The salty-sweet contrast and the interplay of textures create a symphony of flavors that intrigue and delight the taste buds.

2. Hot Chocolate Spice: Chocolate and Hot Sauce

A dash of heat meets the velvety sweetness of chocolate in this surprising union. The spicy kick of hot sauce adds depth and complexity to the familiar indulgence of chocolate, creating a harmonious fusion of sensations.

3. Sweet and Savory Seduction: Potato Chips and Ice Cream

Indulge your taste buds with the salty, crunchy allure of potato chips mingling with the creamy decadence of ice cream. The contrast between the savory chips and the sweet ice cream adds an element of surprise to each bite.

4. Fruity Heat: Watermelon and Tajin

The juicy freshness of watermelon meets the zesty heat of Tajin seasoning in this unexpected combination. The tangy, spicy notes of Tajin enhance the natural sweetness of the watermelon, creating a refreshingly unique taste experience.

The Art of Curated Combinations: A DIY Exploration

The world of wacky cravings is an invitation to become a culinary explorer, a flavor architect who embraces the unconventional and redefines the boundaries of taste. By experimenting with your own curated combinations, you can embark on a journey of taste discovery and create personalized indulgences that speak to your unique preferences.

1. Flavor Fusion: Blend ingredients from different culinary traditions to create unexpected flavor profiles. Try adding a sprinkle of cinnamon to your coffee, a drizzle of honey to your pizza, or a dash of sea salt to your chocolate.

2. Textural Contrasts: Explore combinations that play on textural contrasts. Pair the creaminess of avocado with the crunch of potato chips, or layer smooth nut butter on crispy toast for a satisfying bite.

3. Surprising Synergy: Experiment with ingredients that share surprising synergies. Combine the earthy richness of mushrooms with the sweetness of strawberries, or marry the saltiness of feta cheese with the juiciness of watermelon.

The Joy of Wacky Exploration: Celebrating Culinary Creativity

Wacky cravings are a celebration of culinary creativity, a testament to the endless possibilities that await within the realm of taste. By embracing unconventional pairings and exploring the nuances of flavor, you tap into the joy of discovery and deepen your connection to the world of food.

1. Curiosity and Playfulness: Approaching wacky cravings with curiosity and playfulness allows you to engage your senses fully and experience the joy of unexpected flavor

combinations. Let go of preconceived notions and open yourself to new taste adventures.

2. Mindful Indulgence: Savor each bite mindfully, paying attention to the intricate interplay of flavors and textures. Mindful eating enhances your appreciation of the culinary journey and allows you to fully immerse yourself in the experience.

3. Culinary Conversation: Share your wacky creations with friends and family, sparking conversations and inspiring others to explore unconventional combinations. Culinary exploration becomes a shared adventure that fosters connection and camaraderie.

Conclusion

Wacky cravings transport us to a world of flavor alchemy, where the ordinary becomes extraordinary and the predictable transforms into the unexpected. By embracing the allure of unconventional pairings, we celebrate the versatility of the human palate and the joy of culinary exploration.

In the chapters that follow, we will continue our exploration of the dynamic realm of taste, delve into the impact of societal influences on our culinary preferences, and uncover strategies to cultivate a balanced and mindful approach to eating. As we peel back the layers of taste exploration and culinary creativity, we will gain insight into the mechanisms that shape our indulgences and embark on a journey to reclaim our sense of delight, discovery, and culinary fulfillment. So, dear reader, join us as we revel in the world of wacky cravings and embrace a path toward flavor exploration and self-discovery.

18.
THE PRICE WE PAY: UNRAVELING THE ECONOMIC AND HEALTH COSTS

Junk food, with its alluring flavors and convenient accessibility, has entrenched itself as a staple in modern diets. Yet, beneath the surface of our indulgent cravings lies a complex web of consequences that extend far beyond our taste buds. In this chapter, we delve into the multifaceted landscape of the economic and health costs associated with our love affair with junk food. We will explore the financial toll on individuals and societies, and we'll confront the toll it takes on our well-being, unravelling the intricate ties between our dietary choices and the price we ultimately pay.

Counting the Dollars: Economic Impact of Junk Food

The allure of junk food is not just a matter of taste; it has profound economic implications that ripple through our personal finances and societal systems. As we indulge in convenient and often inexpensive options, we may unwittingly be paying a high price in the long run.

1. Healthcare Costs: The consumption of junk food is linked to a range of health issues, including obesity, diabetes, heart disease, and more. These health conditions place a significant burden on healthcare systems, leading to increased medical costs and reduced quality of life for affected individuals.

2. Productivity Loss: Poor dietary choices can lead to decreased productivity due to increased absenteeism, decreased energy levels, and decreased cognitive function. This productivity loss affects both individuals and workplaces, resulting in economic consequences.

3. Environmental Impact: The production and distribution of junk food contribute to environmental degradation, including deforestation, water pollution, and

greenhouse gas emissions. These environmental costs have far-reaching implications for future generations and global ecosystems.

4. Healthcare Industry Strain: The demand for healthcare services to address diet-related health issues strains healthcare resources and infrastructure. This strain affects the availability and affordability of healthcare for all individuals.

The True Cost of Convenience: Health Implications

While junk food may offer immediate gratification, the long-term health consequences are far from satisfying. The toll it takes on our well-being can be devastating, affecting not only our physical health but also our emotional and mental states.

1. Obesity Epidemic: Junk food is a leading contributor to the obesity epidemic, which is associated with a host of health problems, including diabetes, heart disease, joint issues, and more. The struggle with obesity

places a significant burden on individuals'
health and well-being.

2. Chronic Diseases: The consumption of
excessive sugar, unhealthy fats, and
processed ingredients contributes to the
development of chronic diseases such as
diabetes, hypertension, and cardiovascular
diseases. These conditions lead to
diminished quality of life and increased
mortality rates.

3. Mental Health Impact: Poor dietary choices
have been linked to an increased risk of
mental health disorders, including depression
and anxiety. The gut-brain connection
underscores the importance of a balanced
diet in maintaining emotional well-being.

4. Reduced Longevity: The health
consequences of a diet rich in junk food can
lead to a shorter lifespan, robbing individuals
of precious years of vitality and enjoyment.

Breaking the Cycle: Strategies for Change

The economic and health costs associated
with junk food consumption may seem

overwhelming, but the power to effect change lies within our choices. By taking proactive steps and making informed decisions, we can gradually break free from the cycle of indulgence and its consequences.

1. Education and Awareness: The first step toward change is education and awareness. By understanding the impact of junk food on our health and society, we become better equipped to make informed choices.

2. Balanced Nutrition: Prioritize a balanced and nutrient-rich diet that includes whole foods, fruits, vegetables, lean proteins, and healthy fats. These choices provide essential nutrients that support overall health and well-being.

3. Mindful Eating: Practice mindful eating by savoring each bite, eating slowly, and paying attention to hunger and fullness cues. Mindful eating helps prevent overeating and promotes a healthier relationship with food.

4. Culinary Exploration: Explore new recipes and cooking techniques that prioritize whole, unprocessed ingredients. Engaging in

culinary creativity can make healthy eating enjoyable and satisfying.

5. Policy Advocacy: Support policies and initiatives that promote access to healthy foods and discourage the overconsumption of junk food. Advocacy can contribute to positive changes at the societal level.

Shifting the Paradigm: A Path Forward

The economic and health costs of our indulgence in junk food are stark reminders of the intricate connections between our dietary choices, our well-being, and the larger societal context. As we confront the price we pay for our dietary habits, we are empowered to make choices that promote a healthier and more sustainable future.

In the chapters that follow, we will continue our exploration of the multifaceted landscape of dietary behaviors, delve into the role of cultural influences, and uncover strategies to foster a balanced and mindful approach to eating. As we peel back the layers of economic and health consequences, we will gain insight into the mechanisms that shape our indulgences and embark on a journey to reclaim our sense of agency, well-being, and societal responsibility. So, dear reader, join us as we navigate the complex terrain of economic and health costs and embrace a path toward positive change and self-discovery.

19.
CHEAT DAY CHRONICLES: EPIC BINGES AND THE MORNING AFTER

Ah, the alluring promise of a cheat day – a designated time when dietary restrictions loosen their grip, and we indulge in the forbidden pleasures of our favorite junk foods. It's a day of culinary freedom, a celebration of flavors, and a chance to let our taste buds dance with delight. Yet, as the feast unfolds and the last crumbs are savored, there's a familiar companion waiting in the wings: the morning after. In this chapter, we dive into the world of cheat days, exploring the euphoria of epic binges, the aftermath of indulgence, and the complex interplay of pleasure and regret that accompanies this much-anticipated day.

Embracing the Feast: The Euphoria of Cheat Days

Cheat days are a tantalizing promise that temporarily liberates us from dietary restrictions. It's a day when we indulge in our favorite treats without guilt or hesitation. The anticipation builds, and as the day dawns, we embrace the feast with open arms and eager taste buds.

1. The Pleasure Principle: The allure of cheat days lies in the principle of pleasure. Our taste buds revel in the symphony of flavors, the richness of textures, and the indulgence of our culinary desires. Every bite becomes a moment of sensory celebration, an homage to the joy of eating.

2. Culinary Adventure: Cheat days are an opportunity to embark on a culinary adventure, exploring the foods we've been craving and the ones we've dreamt of trying. It's a day of exploration, where every meal becomes a canvas for flavor experimentation.

3. Mental Break: Beyond the physical indulgence, cheat days offer a mental break from the rigidity of dietary rules. It's a chance to pause, relax, and revel in the freedom to enjoy without restraint. The mental respite

provides a temporary escape from the pressures of maintaining a strict diet.

The Morning After: Navigating Pleasure and Regret

As the feast comes to a close and the clock resets, the morning after arrives. It's a time of reflection, both on the pleasures of the previous day and the potential consequences of indulgence. The interplay of pleasure and regret takes center stage, creating a complex emotional landscape.

1. **The Taste of Regret:** The morning after a cheat day often comes with a tinge of regret. The pleasures of indulgence are replaced by feelings of guilt and self-criticism. The foods that brought us so much joy now become a source of unease, as we grapple with the aftermath of our culinary escapade.

2. **The Physical Effects:** Indulgence can lead to physical discomfort, ranging from bloating and digestive issues to a general sense of lethargy. The body's response to a sudden influx of indulgent foods serves as a reminder

of the impact our dietary choices can have on our well-being.

3. Emotional Turmoil: The morning after is a time of emotional turmoil, where we navigate the conflicting emotions of pleasure and regret. We oscillate between relishing the culinary adventure and chastising ourselves for overindulgence.

The Complex Psychology of Indulgence

The interplay between pleasure and regret on cheat days is a testament to the intricate psychology of indulgence. It reflects the tension between immediate gratification and long-term well-being, between the pursuit of pleasure and the pursuit of health.

1. The Temporal Divide: Cheat days highlight the temporal divide between the immediate pleasure of indulgence and the potential consequences that manifest later. The joy of the moment is juxtaposed with the potential regret that lingers in the aftermath.

2. Emotional Fulfillment: Indulgence often provides a temporary emotional fulfillment,

serving as a source of comfort, celebration, or distraction. However, this emotional fulfillment is fleeting, giving way to a range of emotions as the day transitions into the morning after.

3. The Quest for Balance: The psychology of cheat days underscores the delicate quest for balance – the desire to enjoy indulgence while minimizing its potential negative effects. It reflects the ongoing negotiation between our pleasure-seeking instincts and our health-conscious intentions.

Navigating the Complex Terrain: Strategies for Balance

Navigating the rollercoaster of emotions and sensations that accompany cheat days requires a mindful approach that embraces both pleasure and responsibility. Here are strategies to help you navigate the complex terrain of cheat days and find a sense of balance:

1. Mindful Indulgence: Embrace mindful eating on cheat days by savoring each bite and fully engaging your senses. Mindful indulgence allows you to experience the pleasures of your favorite treats without losing sight of the present moment.

2. Moderation: While cheat days offer a chance to indulge, moderation remains key. Opt for smaller portions, share treats with loved ones, or choose a few indulgences that truly bring you joy.

3. Self-Compassion: Practice self-compassion and kindness, both during and after cheat days. Acknowledge the pleasures of indulgence without harsh self-judgment. Remember that one day of indulgence does not define your overall dietary journey.

4. Balanced Recovery: The morning after is an opportunity for balanced recovery. Prioritize hydration, choose nutrient-rich foods, and engage in gentle physical activity to support your body's transition back to regular eating patterns.

5. Learn and Adjust: Reflect on your cheat day experiences to gain insight into your emotional and physical responses. Use this information to adjust your approach for future

cheat days, finding a balance that works for you.

Conclusion

Cheat days are a nuanced dance of pleasure and responsibility, an exploration of indulgence and its consequences. As we embrace the feast and navigate the morning after, we gain a deeper understanding of the psychology of indulgence and the intricate ties between pleasure, regret, and well-being.

In the chapters that follow, we will continue our exploration of the complex landscape of dietary behaviors, delve into the role of societal influences, and uncover strategies to foster a balanced and mindful approach to eating. As we peel back the layers of pleasure and responsibility, we will gain insight into the mechanisms that shape our indulgences and embark on a journey to reclaim our sense of enjoyment, self-awareness, and culinary fulfillment. So, dear reader, join us as we journey through the world of cheat days and embrace a path toward balance and self-discovery.

20.
THE ART OF MODERATION: FINDING BALANCE IN A JUNK FOOD WORLD

In a world saturated with enticing junk food options, finding balance can seem like an elusive pursuit. The allure of indulgence and the pressures of health-consciousness create a constant tug-of-war within us. In this chapter, we delve into the delicate art of moderation – a skill that empowers us to navigate the tempting landscape of junk food while maintaining a sense of equilibrium. We will explore the principles of moderation, uncover strategies for cultivating this art, and embrace the wisdom of harmonizing pleasure and well-being in a world of culinary temptation.

The Quest for Balance: The Essence of Moderation

Moderation is the cornerstone of a harmonious relationship with junk food. It's not about deprivation or strict rules; rather, it's a conscious and intentional approach to enjoying indulgences without losing sight of overall health and well-being. The quest for balance requires a blend of self-awareness, mindfulness, and a commitment to nourishing both the body and the soul.

1. Mindful Consumption: Moderation begins with mindful consumption. It involves savoring each bite, fully engaging the senses, and being present in the moment. Mindful eating allows us to appreciate the flavors and textures of our indulgences without mindlessly overindulging.

2. Listening to Hunger and Fullness: Paying attention to hunger and fullness cues is a fundamental aspect of moderation. By tuning into our body's signals, we can make informed choices about when to indulge and when to stop, ensuring that we satisfy cravings without overdoing it.

3. Quality over Quantity: Moderation prioritizes quality over quantity. Instead of

mindlessly consuming large quantities of junk food, focus on savoring small portions of high-quality treats. This approach allows you to fully enjoy the experience without sacrificing well-being.

4. **Variety and Balance:** Embrace variety in your dietary choices to foster a balanced approach. Incorporate a diverse range of nutrient-rich foods alongside occasional indulgences. This balance ensures that your overall nutritional needs are met while allowing room for treats.

The Paradox of Pleasure and Restraint

Moderation dances at the intersection of pleasure and restraint, embodying the paradoxical nature of our relationship with junk food. It recognizes the joy that indulgence brings while advocating for self-control and conscious decision-making.

1. **Pleasure Without Guilt:** Moderation reframes indulgence as a source of pleasure rather than guilt. It allows us to relish the flavors and experiences of junk food without

the burden of remorse, fostering a healthier emotional relationship with treats.

2. Mindful Choice: The art of moderation involves making mindful choices. It's about consciously deciding when and how to indulge, rather than succumbing to impulsive cravings. This practice empowers us to be in control of our choices and align them with our well-being goals.

3. Self-Discipline: Embracing moderation requires a degree of self-discipline. It's about acknowledging cravings while also recognizing the importance of maintaining a balanced and nourishing diet. Self-discipline allows us to find a middle ground between unrestrained indulgence and rigid restriction.

Strategies for Cultivating Moderation

Cultivating the art of moderation is a skill that can be honed over time. By implementing practical strategies and adopting a mindful approach, you can navigate the world of junk food with greater ease and confidence.

1. **Plan Ahead**: Set intentions and plan for indulgences in advance. Knowing when and how you'll enjoy treats helps you approach them mindfully and prevents impulsive overindulgence.

2. **Portion Control**: Practice portion control by selecting smaller serving sizes of indulgent foods. Savor each bite and focus on quality rather than quantity.

3. **Mindful Eating**: Engage in mindful eating by paying attention to the sensory experience of eating. Chew slowly, savor the flavors, and listen to your body's signals of hunger and fullness.

4. **Occasional Indulgences**: Treat junk food as occasional indulgences rather than everyday staples. This approach allows you to enjoy them without compromising your overall well-being.

5. **Balanced Lifestyle**: Embrace a balanced lifestyle that includes regular physical activity, stress management, and ample sleep. A holistic approach to well-being supports your ability to make mindful choices.

Embracing the Art of Moderation: A Path to Harmony

The art of moderation is a journey of self-discovery and empowerment. It's a path that encourages us to find harmony between our desires and our well-being, between pleasure and responsibility.

1. Self-Awareness: Develop self-awareness by tuning into your cravings, triggers, and emotional responses. Understanding your relationship with food allows you to make conscious choices that align with your goals.

2. Flexibility and Forgiveness: Embrace flexibility in your approach to eating. Allow for occasional indulgences without attaching guilt. Practice self-forgiveness when you veer off course and use setbacks as opportunities for learning.

3. Joyful Eating: Embrace the joy of eating and celebrate the pleasures that food brings to your life. Allow yourself to savor the experience, knowing that you can enjoy treats without sacrificing your overall well-being.

4. Long-Term Sustainability: Recognize that moderation is a sustainable approach to your dietary choices. It's not a short-term fix but a lifelong commitment to finding balance and nourishing both your body and your soul.

Mindful Evolution: The art of moderation evolves as you do. Your preferences, needs, and priorities may change over time, and that's perfectly okay. Adapt your approach to suit your current circumstances and continue to prioritize your well-being.

Conclusion:

A Journey of Flavor and Wisdom

As we conclude our exploration of the delicate art of moderation, we stand at the crossroads of pleasure and well-being, armed with insights and strategies to navigate the enticing world of junk food. The journey of moderation is not about rigidity or sacrifice; rather, it's an invitation to engage with the flavors of life mindfully and intentionally.

In the chapters that have preceded this one, we've delved into the enticing allure of junk food, uncovered the science of cravings, examined the impact of marketing, and explored the transformative power of redemption. Now, as we embrace the art of moderation, we extend an invitation to you, dear reader, to embark on a path of mindful consumption and balanced indulgence.

May your culinary journey be guided by self-awareness, pleasure, and a deep appreciation for the flavors that enrich your life. As you savor each bite, may you find harmony in the interplay of indulgence and restraint, and may the art of moderation empower you to forge a sustainable and nourishing relationship with the culinary world around you.

With this chapter, we bid adieu to our exploration of "The Crap We Consume." Yet, the wisdom and insights gathered throughout our journey will remain with us, serving as beacons of guidance as we navigate the landscapes of taste, desire, and well-being. So, dear reader, may your path be one of mindful choices, delightful indulgences, and a vibrant celebration of the art of moderation.

21.

CELEBRITY INDULGENCES: WHAT A-LISTERS REALLY SNACK ON

Celebrities: they're just like us... or are they? While we often associate A-listers with their glamorous lifestyles and seemingly flawless physiques, the truth is that even the rich and famous have their own guilty pleasures. In this chapter, we pull back the curtain on celebrity snacking habits, shedding light on the indulgent treats that even Hollywood's elite can't resist. From quirky combinations to unexpected cravings, we explore the human side of these larger-than-life figures and uncover the surprising world of celebrity indulgences.

Behind the Scenes: The Myth of Perfection

Celebrities are often portrayed as paragons of health and beauty, with their seemingly flawless appearances and disciplined lifestyles. However, the reality is more complex than the polished images we see on the screen. Like all of us, celebrities have their moments of weakness, their cravings, and their indulgent escapes from the pressures of stardom.

1. Humanizing the Stars: Understanding the indulgent snacking habits of celebrities humanizes them and reminds us that, at the end of the day, they're just ordinary people with extraordinary careers. Their indulgences connect them to the universal experience of seeking comfort and pleasure through food.

2. The Myth of Perfection: Celebrity indulgences shatter the myth of perfection, revealing that even those who seem to have it all struggle with the same cravings and desires that we do. This realization encourages a more compassionate and relatable view of these iconic figures.

Quirky Combinations and Guilty Pleasures

From extravagant treats to unexpected cravings, celebrities offer a glimpse into their snacking habits that often defy expectations. These indulgences showcase the diversity of tastes and preferences that make each celebrity unique.

1. Sweet and Savory: Some celebrities gravitate toward the combination of sweet and savory, such as Dwayne "The Rock" Johnson, who is known to enjoy stacks of pancakes topped with peanut butter and syrup. This quirky pairing captures the interplay of flavors that can tantalize the taste buds.

2. Comfort Classics: Many A-listers find solace in comfort classics that remind them of their childhood or simpler times. Oprah Winfrey's love for mashed potatoes and Drew Barrymore's affection for grilled cheese sandwiches reflect a yearning for familiar and comforting flavors.

3. Healthier Indulgences: While indulgent, some celebrity choices align with a health-conscious approach. Jennifer Aniston's fondness for dark chocolate and Cameron Diaz's preference for avocado toast

demonstrate that even indulgence can be tailored to healthier options.

The Influence of Culture and Tradition

Celebrities often reflect the cultural and traditional influences that shape their snacking preferences. These influences provide insight into their backgrounds and heritage, offering a deeper understanding of their culinary choices.

1. Global Flavors: A-listers with diverse backgrounds bring a tapestry of global flavors to their indulgences. Priyanka Chopra's love for samosas and Chrissy Teigen's affinity for Filipino dishes like lumpia showcase the fusion of cultures that shape their palates.

2. Nostalgia and Heritage: For some celebrities, indulgences are rooted in nostalgia and heritage. Beyoncé's enjoyment of Southern comfort foods like fried chicken and Jay-Z's love for New York-style pizza reflect the connections between food, identity, and upbringing.

Balancing Indulgence and Wellness

Celebrity indulgences offer a snapshot of the ongoing struggle to balance pleasure with wellness. Like all of us, A-listers strive to find equilibrium in their dietary choices, sometimes opting for indulgence and at other times prioritizing nourishment.

1. Mindful Choices: Some celebrities approach indulgence mindfully, making conscious choices to enjoy treats while also taking care of their bodies. Reese Witherspoon's moderation in treating herself to favorite desserts exemplifies this approach.

2. Occasional Splurges: Many celebrities view indulgences as occasional splurges that add richness to their lives. Heidi Klum's affection for German pastries and Katy Perry's love for In-N-Out burgers demonstrate how these treats punctuate their healthy routines.

3. Balance and Self-Care: Celebrity indulgences underscore the importance of balance and self-care. By incorporating occasional indulgences into their lives, A-listers embrace a well-rounded approach to

wellness that includes both physical nourishment and emotional satisfaction.

Celebrity Indulgences: A Lesson in Humanity

The snacking habits of celebrities offer more than just a glimpse into their personal lives; they provide a lesson in humanity, reminding us that indulgence and pleasure are universal experiences that connect us all.

1. Celebrating Diversity: Celebrity indulgences celebrate the diversity of tastes and preferences that define our culinary identities. They remind us that no matter our backgrounds or status, we all seek comfort, pleasure, and joy through food.

2. Challenging Stereotypes: The indulgences of A-listers challenge stereotypes and showcase the complexity of human nature. These choices reveal that even those who seem larger than life grapple with the same desires and cravings as everyone else.

3. Embracing Imperfection: Celebrity indulgences encourage us to embrace imperfection and let go of the pursuit of

flawless living. They remind us that indulgence is a part of a well-rounded and fulfilling life, and that finding joy in treats is an essential aspect of our shared human experience.

Conclusion

In the world of celebrities, indulgences offer a window into the authenticity and relatability that often lie beneath the glitz and glamour. As we uncover the surprising snacking habits of A-listers, we gain a deeper appreciation for the complexity of human desires and the universal need for pleasure and comfort.

In the chapters that follow, we will continue our exploration of the multifaceted landscape of dietary behaviors, delve into the role of societal influences, and uncover strategies to foster a balanced and mindful approach to eating. As we peel back the layers of celebrity indulgences, we will gain insight into the mechanisms that shape our indulgences and embark on a journey to reclaim our sense of pleasure, authenticity, and culinary fulfillment. So, dear reader, join us as we journey through the world of celebrity snacking and embrace a path toward self-discovery and harmony.

22.

JUNK FOOD HACKS: TRICKS TO SATISFY CRAVINGS WITHOUT GOING OVERBOARD

Junk food cravings are a universal experience, tempting us with their irresistible allure. Yet, succumbing to these cravings doesn't have to mean diving headfirst into a sea of indulgence. In this chapter, we uncover a treasure trove of junk food hacks – clever strategies and creative alternatives that allow you to satisfy your cravings without losing sight of your health and well-being. From mindful substitutions to portion control tricks, we explore the art of indulgence in a way that promotes balance and mindful enjoyment.

Cravings Unleashed: The Power of Temptation

Junk food cravings are a force to be reckoned with, often triggered by a combination of sensory cues, emotions, and psychological factors. Understanding the power of cravings is the first step in learning how to manage them effectively.

1. The Sensory Experience: Cravings are often triggered by the sensory allure of junk food – the sight, smell, and taste that instantly transport us to a realm of pleasure. Visual cues and aromas play a significant role in igniting our desire for indulgence.

2. Emotional Triggers: Emotions play a pivotal role in cravings, with stress, boredom, and sadness often fueling our desire for comfort foods. Emotional eating can lead to mindless indulgence, as we seek solace in familiar treats.

3. Psychological Associations: Cravings are also shaped by psychological associations we've developed over time. Certain foods become linked to positive memories or experiences, reinforcing our inclination to turn to them for comfort or pleasure.

Mindful Indulgence: The Art of Satisfaction

Mindful indulgence is about finding the sweet spot between satisfying your cravings and maintaining a sense of balance. By applying mindful strategies, you can navigate the landscape of junk food temptations with intention and awareness.

1. **Pause and Reflect:** When a craving strikes, take a moment to pause and reflect. Ask yourself if you're truly hungry or if there's an emotional trigger at play. Mindful awareness helps you differentiate between genuine hunger and a desire for comfort.

2. **Savor the Moment:** If you decide to indulge, do so mindfully. Savor each bite, paying attention to the flavors, textures, and sensations. Mindful eating enhances the pleasure of indulgence and prevents mindless overconsumption.

3. **One-Bite Bliss:** Sometimes, all it takes is a single bite to satisfy a craving. Allow yourself to enjoy a small portion of the desired treat, relishing the initial burst of flavor. Often, this bite is enough to quell the craving's intensity.

Smart Swaps and Creative Alternatives

Junk food hacks often involve clever substitutions and creative alternatives that allow you to enjoy the flavors you crave while making healthier choices.

1. Ingredient Substitutions: Experiment with ingredient substitutions to create healthier versions of your favorite junk foods. Replace refined flour with whole grains, use natural sweeteners in place of processed sugars, and incorporate nutrient-dense ingredients.

2. DIY Delights: Make your own junk food favorites at home using quality ingredients. Bake homemade cookies, air-pop your popcorn, or create your version of savory chips using vegetables like kale or sweet potatoes.

3. Portion Control Tricks: Trick your brain by using smaller plates and bowls for indulgent snacks. A smaller serving size can create the illusion of a satisfying portion while reducing overall consumption.

The Art of Distraction and Delay

Sometimes, managing cravings is about redirecting your attention and delaying gratification. These techniques give you time to assess whether the craving is genuine or a passing desire.

1. Engage in Activities: When a craving hits, engage in an activity that captures your attention and shifts your focus away from food. Take a walk, practice a hobby, or engage in a brief workout to redirect your energy.

2. Time-Based Delay: Give yourself a time-based delay before indulging in a craving. Set a timer for 10-15 minutes and engage in another activity. Often, the initial intensity of the craving subsides during this time.

3. Drink Water: Drinking a glass of water before succumbing to a craving can help reduce its intensity. Sometimes, our bodies confuse thirst with hunger, and hydration can satisfy the urge.

The Power of Mindset: Cultivating Self-Awareness

Mindset plays a crucial role in managing junk food cravings. By cultivating self-awareness and adopting a balanced perspective, you can develop a healthier relationship with indulgence.

1. Remove Judgment: Approach cravings without judgment. Acknowledge that cravings are a natural part of being human and don't define your worth or self-control.

2. Practice Compassion: Be kind to yourself, whether you choose to indulge or make a healthier choice. Self-compassion helps you navigate the ebb and flow of cravings without resorting to guilt or shame.

3. Reflect and Learn: After indulging, take time to reflect on the experience. What triggered the craving? How did you feel before and after indulgence? Learning from each experience can help you make more mindful choices in the future.

Conclusion

Junk food hacks empower you to navigate the world of cravings with creativity, intention, and self-awareness. By applying mindful strategies, making smart swaps, and adopting a balanced mindset, you can satisfy your indulgent desires without compromising your overall well-being.

In the chapters that follow, we will continue our exploration of the multifaceted landscape of dietary behaviors, delve into the role of societal influences, and uncover strategies to foster a balanced and mindful approach to eating. As we peel back the layers of junk food indulgence, we will gain insight into the mechanisms that shape our cravings and embark on a journey to reclaim our sense of empowerment, satisfaction, and culinary fulfillment. So, dear reader, join us as we unravel the world of junk food hacks and embrace a path toward self-discovery and mindful enjoyment.

23.

FROM TRASH TO TREASURE: UPCYCLING JUNK FOOD FOR CULINARY CREATIVITY

What if the remnants of your indulgent snack session could be transformed into a masterpiece of culinary creativity? In this chapter, we embark on a journey from trash to treasure, exploring the art of upcycling junk food. By repurposing leftover treats and forgotten goodies, we unlock a realm of gastronomic innovation that breathes new life into familiar flavors. From decadent desserts to savory delights, we dive into the world of upcycled culinary creations that bridge the gap between indulgence and ingenuity.

From Indulgence to Inspiration: The Concept of Upcycling

Upcycling is the art of transforming discarded or unused items into something of greater value. When it comes to junk food, upcycling takes on a delicious twist as we reimagine leftover treats as ingredients for culinary exploration.

1. Repurposing Indulgence: Upcycling junk food is about turning indulgent snacks into a source of culinary inspiration. It challenges us to view these treats not only as end-of-day indulgences but also as potential building blocks for innovative dishes.

2. Reducing Food Waste: Upcycling aligns with the goal of reducing food waste, a significant issue in modern society. By repurposing leftover junk food, we contribute to a more sustainable culinary approach.

3. Creative Fusion: Upcycling is a form of creative fusion, combining the familiar flavors of junk food with unexpected ingredients to craft unique and memorable dishes.

Sweet Concoctions: Dessert Transformations

Junk food desserts become the canvas for upcycling, where imagination takes center stage and new dimensions of flavor are unveiled.

1. Cookie Crumbles: Leftover cookies find new purpose as crumbles for pies, tarts, and ice cream toppings. Their texture and sweetness add depth to a variety of desserts.

2. Candy Capers: Unwanted candies become vibrant garnishes for cakes, cupcakes, and sundaes. Melted down, they can be transformed into colorful drizzles or swirls.

3. Chocolate Makeover: Excess chocolate bars can be melted and repurposed as decadent fondue or used as a base for homemade hot chocolate.

Savory Sensations: Reinventing Leftovers

The world of upcycling extends to savory creations, where leftover chips, crackers, and other salty indulgences take on new roles in the culinary realm.

1. Crispy Coatings: Crushed chips or crackers serve as creative coatings for chicken tenders, fish fillets, or roasted vegetables, adding crunch and flavor.

2. Breading Bliss: Processed snack crumbs act as a unique breading for dishes like chicken nuggets or mozzarella sticks, infusing them with a hint of familiar flavor.

3. Flavorful Fillings: Leftover cheese puffs or pretzels can be ground into fillings for stuffed peppers, mushrooms, or dumplings, imparting an unexpected twist.

Mastering the Art: Tips for Successful Upcycling

Upcycling junk food requires a mix of culinary know-how, experimentation, and a dash of creativity. Here are tips to guide you on your upcycling journey.

1. Flavor Pairing: Consider the flavor profiles of your junk food ingredients and pair them with complementary flavors to create harmonious and balanced dishes.

2. Texture Play: Explore how the textures of your upcycled ingredients can add dimension to your creations. Crunchy crumbs, creamy fillings, and gooey centers all contribute to a delightful eating experience.

3. Recipe Adaptation: Adapt existing recipes by incorporating upcycled ingredients as substitutes or enhancements. Be open to experimenting and adjusting proportions to achieve the desired results.

4. Presentation Matters: Elevate the visual appeal of your upcycled dishes through creative plating and garnishes. A well-presented dish enhances the overall dining experience.

5. Celebrate Creativity: Embrace the playful and imaginative nature of upcycling. There's no right or wrong – only the joy of experimentation and the thrill of culinary discovery.

The Joy of Culinary Alchemy

Upcycling junk food is a form of culinary alchemy, where discarded treasures are transformed into gastronomic wonders. It invites us to step outside the confines of traditional recipes and embrace a world of innovation and possibility.

1. A Journey of Exploration: Upcycling junk food is a journey of exploration, where the unexpected becomes a source of inspiration. It encourages us to push culinary boundaries and venture into uncharted territory.

2. Embracing Imperfection: Upcycling celebrates imperfection and embraces the quirky charm of unconventional combinations. It's a reminder that culinary brilliance often emerges from the most unexpected sources.

3. Culinary Sustainability: The practice of upcycling aligns with the principles of culinary sustainability, promoting resourcefulness and minimizing food waste. It's a small but impactful way to contribute to a more sustainable food system.

Conclusion

From trash to treasure, upcycling junk food invites us to reimagine the possibilities that lie within our indulgent treats. It's a celebration of culinary creativity, a dance between indulgence and innovation that transforms forgotten goodies into culinary marvels.

In the chapters that follow, we will continue our exploration of the multifaceted landscape of dietary behaviors, delve into the role of societal influences, and uncover strategies to foster a balanced and mindful approach to eating. As we peel back the layers of upcycled culinary creations, we will gain insight into the mechanisms that shape our culinary ingenuity and embark on a journey to reclaim our sense of creativity, experimentation, and culinary fulfillment. So, dear reader, join us as we dive into the world of upcycling junk food and embrace a path toward gastronomic exploration and self-discovery.

24.

ICONIC EATS: LEGENDARY JUNK FOOD ITEMS THAT SHAPED A GENERATION

Junk food isn't just about flavors and indulgence – it's also a cultural phenomenon that has left an indelible mark on generations. In this chapter, we embark on a nostalgic journey through time, exploring the legendary junk food items that have shaped the culinary landscape and captured the hearts (and taste buds) of millions. From iconic snacks that sparked childhood memories to treats that defined an era, we delve into the stories behind these beloved edibles and uncover the cultural impact they've had on society.

Culinary Nostalgia: The Power of Iconic Junk Food

Iconic junk food items hold a special place in our hearts, often evoking fond memories and a sense of nostalgia. These treats go beyond mere consumption – they become symbols of shared experiences and cultural touchstones.

1. Cultural Icons: Iconic junk food items are cultural icons that transcend their status as snacks. They become woven into the fabric of society, reflecting the trends, tastes, and values of their respective eras.

2. Emotional Connections: These treats forge emotional connections that span generations. The taste of a childhood favorite can transport us back in time, evoking feelings of comfort, joy, and nostalgia.

3. Shared Experiences: Iconic junk food items create shared experiences that bring people together. Whether enjoyed at parties, movie nights, or after-school hangouts, these treats facilitate moments of connection and camaraderie.

Snack Time Stories: Legendary Junk Food Items

From classic chips to sweet confections, legendary junk food items have become synonymous with certain eras and cultural shifts.

1. **Doritos:** Introduced in the 1960s, Doritos revolutionized the snack scene with their bold and flavorful tortilla chips. Their success marked a shift towards more adventurous and daring snack choices.

2. **Twinkies:** The Twinkie, born in the 1930s, became a symbol of American ingenuity and resilience. Its enduring popularity has made it a beloved treat that has stood the test of time.

3. **Pop Rocks:** The fizzy, popping sensation of Pop Rocks candy captured the imagination of the 1970s generation, showcasing the thrill of unexpected flavor experiences.

4. **Snack Cakes:** Snack cakes like Hostess CupCakes and Ding Dongs became lunchbox staples and after-school delights, embodying the simple pleasures of childhood snacking.

5. Jell-O Pudding Pops: These frozen treats, endorsed by Bill Cosby in the 1980s, epitomized the allure of convenience and indulgence.

Cultural Shifts and Societal Impact

The rise of iconic junk food items often mirrors larger cultural shifts and societal changes.

1. The Rise of Convenience: Iconic junk food items are often associated with the growing demand for convenience in modern life. These snacks catered to busy schedules and the desire for instant gratification.

2. Advertising and Branding: The success of legendary junk food items was often fueled by clever advertising and memorable branding. Slogans, mascots, and jingles became embedded in popular culture.

3. The Influence of Pop Culture: Iconic junk food items were featured in movies, TV shows, and music, further cementing their place in the cultural zeitgeist. They became symbols of a certain era's popular culture.

Legacy and Nostalgia

The legacy of iconic junk food items lives on, leaving an imprint that extends beyond their original release.

1. **Nostalgia's Pull:** The nostalgia associated with legendary junk food items continues to draw consumers back to these treats, creating a sense of comfort and familiarity.

2. **Resurgence and Revival:** Some iconic junk food items experience resurgences, with brands capitalizing on their nostalgic appeal by reintroducing them to new generations.

3. **Cultural Conversations:** Legendary junk food items often spark cultural conversations, inviting discussions about changing tastes, nostalgia, and the evolution of culinary preferences.

Conclusion

Iconic junk food items are more than just snacks – they're cultural touchstones, time capsules that capture the essence of a generation. As we journey through the stories behind these legendary treats, we gain a deeper appreciation for the role they've played in shaping our collective culinary identity and cultural landscape.

In the chapters that follow, we will continue our exploration of the multifaceted landscape of dietary behaviors, delve into the role of societal influences, and uncover strategies to foster a balanced and mindful approach to eating. As we peel back the layers of iconic junk food items, we will gain insight into the mechanisms that shape our culinary preferences and embark on a journey to reconnect with the flavors, memories, and cultural significance that make these treats truly legendary. So, dear reader, join us as we dive into the world of iconic eats and embrace a path toward understanding, appreciation, and culinary enrichment.

25.

THE ROAD TO REDEMPTION: INSPIRING TALES OF JUNK FOOD TURNAROUNDS

The journey from junk food indulgence to redemption is a path filled with challenges, resilience, and transformation. In this chapter, we delve into the inspiring tales of individuals who have embarked on the road to redemption – stories of those who have turned their relationship with junk food around, reclaiming their health, vitality, and well-being. Through determination, self-discovery, and perseverance, these individuals have harnessed the power of change to reshape their lives and inspire others on their own paths to redemption.

Facing the Abyss: The Wake-Up Call

For many, the decision to embark on a journey of redemption comes after a significant wake-up call – a moment that prompts a deep realization of the impact of junk food on their health and well-being.

1. Health Crisis: Health crises, such as obesity, diabetes, or heart disease, often serve as wake-up calls that force individuals to confront the consequences of their dietary choices.

2. Personal Reflection: Self-reflection and introspection can lead to the recognition that patterns of junk food consumption are hindering overall well-being and quality of life.

3. External Triggers: External events, such as the birth of a child or the desire to set a positive example for loved ones, can motivate individuals to seek redemption by transforming their relationship with junk food.

The Transformational Journey: Overcoming Challenges

The journey from junk food indulgence to redemption is not without its hurdles. It requires perseverance, resilience, and a commitment to change.

1. Breaking Habits: Overcoming ingrained habits and behaviors is a central challenge on the road to redemption. Individuals must rewire their relationship with food, replacing unhealthy patterns with mindful choices.

2. Emotional Resilience: Addressing emotional eating and developing healthier coping mechanisms are essential aspects of the transformational journey. Confronting underlying emotional triggers is a pivotal step toward redemption.

3. Seeking Support: Many individuals find success by seeking support from health professionals, therapists, or support groups. Building a network of encouragement and guidance can be a lifeline on the path to redemption.

Embracing Change: Strategies for Success

Successful redemption stories are rooted in the adoption of strategies that foster lasting change and promote a balanced relationship with food.

1. Nutritional Education: Educating oneself about the nutritional content of foods and the impact of junk food on health is a foundational step toward making informed dietary choices.

2. Mindful Eating: Embracing mindful eating practices, such as paying attention to hunger and fullness cues, savoring each bite, and avoiding distractions, helps individuals develop a healthier relationship with food.

3. Meal Planning and Preparation: Planning and preparing meals in advance empowers individuals to make mindful choices and avoid impulsive junk food indulgences.

4. Cultivating Joy: Rediscovering the joy of cooking, exploring new recipes, and experimenting with wholesome ingredients can rekindle a passion for food that aligns with health and well-being.

Triumph and Inspiration: The Redemption Story

The journey to redemption is marked by triumphs and moments of inspiration that reinforce the path of positive change.

1. Physical Transformations: Achieving weight loss, improved energy levels, and enhanced overall health serve as tangible rewards that inspire individuals to continue their journey of redemption.

2. Mental Empowerment: Overcoming junk food addiction instills a sense of mental empowerment and resilience, boosting self-confidence and self-esteem.

3. Inspiring Others: Sharing personal redemption stories can inspire others to embark on their own transformative journeys. Becoming a source of inspiration motivates individuals to stay committed to their path.

Legacy and Empowerment

The stories of redemption serve as beacons of hope, demonstrating the potential for positive change and personal growth.

1. Ripple Effect: Individual stories of redemption create a ripple effect, inspiring friends, family members, and even entire communities to make healthier choices and seek their own paths to transformation.

2. Shaping Culture: The collective impact of redemption stories contributes to shifts in cultural norms and attitudes toward food, fostering a greater emphasis on mindful eating and well-being.

3. Embracing Imperfection: Redemption stories remind us that the journey is not linear, and setbacks are a natural part of the process. Embracing imperfection and learning from challenges are essential aspects of the road to redemption.

Conclusion

The road to redemption is a testament to the human capacity for change, growth, and transformation. Through the inspiring tales of those who have turned their relationship with junk food around, we gain a deeper appreciation for the power of determination, resilience, and self-discovery. As we journey through these stories, we are reminded that redemption is not a destination but a continuous journey of self-improvement and empowerment.

In the chapters that follow, we will continue our exploration of the multifaceted landscape of dietary behaviors, delve into the role of societal influences, and uncover strategies to foster a balanced and mindful approach to eating. As we peel back the layers of redemption stories, we will gain insight into the mechanisms that shape our relationship with junk food and embark on a journey of self-transformation and empowerment. So, dear reader, join us as we celebrate the triumphs of those who have walked the road to redemption and embrace a path toward positive change, resilience, and well-being.

26.

BEYOND THE WRAPPER: UNMASKING THE TRUE CULPRITS BEHIND OUR CRAVINGS

Junk food cravings often seem like a mystery, leaving us wondering why we're drawn to certain flavors and textures. In this chapter, we delve beneath the surface to unmask the true culprits behind our cravings. From physiological triggers to emotional cues, we explore the intricate web of factors that influence our desire for junk food. By gaining a deeper understanding of these underlying forces, we can empower ourselves to make more informed choices and cultivate a healthier relationship with indulgence.

The Complex Craving Equation

Cravings are the result of a complex interplay between various physiological, psychological, and environmental factors.

1. **Biochemical Signals:** Hormones and neurotransmitters, such as dopamine and serotonin, play a crucial role in cravings. These chemicals influence mood, pleasure, and appetite, driving us to seek comfort in familiar tastes.

2. **Taste and Texture:** The taste and texture of junk food activate our sensory receptors, triggering pleasure centers in the brain. Crunchy, creamy, sweet, and salty sensations all contribute to the allure of indulgence.

3. **Emotional Associations:** Cravings often stem from emotional associations we've formed over time. Certain foods become linked to memories, events, or feelings, leading us to seek them out for comfort or escape.

The Role of Habit and Routine

Habitual behaviors and routines can greatly influence our cravings and consumption patterns.

1. Neural Pathways: Repetition strengthens neural pathways associated with specific foods. Regular consumption of junk food reinforces these pathways, making cravings more automatic and ingrained.

2. Contextual Triggers: Environmental cues, such as seeing a certain place or hearing a familiar sound, can activate cravings by triggering associations with past indulgences.

3. Routine Rituals: Engaging in consistent routines, such as snacking during a specific time of day or while watching TV, can create a conditioned response that leads to cravings.

Stress, Emotions, and Coping Mechanisms

Emotional triggers and stress play a significant role in driving cravings for comfort foods.

1. Stress Hormones: Stress activates the release of cortisol, which can lead to cravings for sugary and fatty foods that provide quick energy and comfort.

2. Emotional Coping: Emotional eating offers a temporary escape from stress, sadness, or boredom. The act of consuming familiar treats becomes a way to manage emotional turmoil.

3. Pleasure and Dopamine: Indulging in junk food can trigger the release of dopamine, a neurotransmitter associated with pleasure and reward. This neurological response reinforces the connection between indulgence and feeling better.

The Influence of Advertising and Social Norms

External influences, such as advertising and societal norms, shape our perceptions of food and contribute to cravings.

1. Advertising Impact: Clever marketing strategies create associations between junk

food and positive emotions or experiences, driving us to seek out those products.

2. Social Acceptance: Societal norms and peer influence can shape our cravings. When junk food is portrayed as a social activity or a way to fit in, it becomes more appealing.

3. Availability and Accessibility: The ubiquity of junk food in our environment makes it a convenient and accessible option, increasing the likelihood of craving-driven consumption.

Cultivating Awareness and Mindful Choices

Unmasking the true culprits behind our cravings empowers us to make more mindful choices and develop a healthier relationship with indulgence.

1. Self-Awareness: Cultivating self-awareness allows us to recognize the physiological, emotional, and environmental factors that drive our cravings. By understanding these triggers, we can respond with intention rather than impulsivity.

2. Mindful Consumption: Practicing mindful eating involves savoring each bite, paying attention to hunger and fullness cues, and acknowledging the sensory experience of indulgence.

3. Emotional Regulation: Developing alternative coping mechanisms for managing emotions, such as engaging in physical activity, practicing deep breathing, or seeking social support, reduces the reliance on food for emotional comfort.

4. Advertising Literacy: Becoming aware of advertising tactics and recognizing when we're being influenced by marketing can help us make more informed choices and resist the pull of cravings.

Shifting Perspectives: Empowerment and Freedom

Understanding the multifaceted nature of cravings empowers us to take control of our choices and navigate the world of indulgence with greater awareness.

1. Empowered Choices: Armed with knowledge, we can make choices that align with our well-being and values. We can opt for healthier alternatives or indulge mindfully, free from the grip of automatic cravings.

2. Breaking Patterns: By disrupting habitual behaviors and routines, we can weaken the neural pathways associated with cravings, creating space for new, healthier patterns.

3. Emotional Resilience: Developing emotional resilience and coping mechanisms reduces the reliance on food for emotional comfort, giving us the tools to face stress and emotions head-on.

Conclusion

Unmasking the true culprits behind our cravings unveils the intricate web of factors that influence our desire for junk food. As we unravel the complex craving equation, we gain a deeper appreciation for the role of physiology, psychology, and environment in shaping our indulgence-driven behaviors.

In the chapters that follow, we will continue our exploration of the multifaceted landscape of dietary behaviors, delve into the role of societal influences, and uncover strategies to foster a balanced and mindful approach to eating. As we peel back the layers of craving triggers, we will gain insight into the mechanisms that shape our desires and embark on a journey to reclaim our sense of empowerment, awareness, and culinary freedom. So, dear reader, join us as we demystify the true culprits behind our cravings and embrace a path toward mindful consumption and well-being.

27.

BONUS CHAPTER: 5 WEEK BODY TRANSFORMATION, DETOX AND WEIGHT LOSS

Creating a comprehensive 5-week body transformation and weight loss plan requires careful consideration of individual needs, goals, and health status. It's important to consult with a healthcare professional before making any significant changes to your diet or exercise routine. That said, here's a general outline of a 5-week plan that incorporates intermittent fasting and exercises. Remember, this is a sample plan and should be tailored to your specific circumstances.

Week 1 - Preparation and Adjustment:
Note: During the first week, focus on adjusting to the new routine and making gradual changes.
Intermittent Fasting (IF): 16/8 method (16 hours fasting, 8 hours eating)
Day 1-7:

Day 1: Introduce intermittent fasting. Start fasting at 8 PM and break your fast at 12 PM the next day.
Days 2-7: Gradually extend your fasting window by 1 hour each day until you reach 16/8.
Exercise:
Days 1, 3, 5: 30-minute brisk walk or light jog.
Days 2, 4, 6: Bodyweight exercises (push-ups, squats, lunges, planks) - 3 sets of 10-12 reps each.

Week 2 - Stepping Up:

Intermittent Fasting (IF): 16/8 method
Days 8-14:
Days 8-14: Continue with the 16/8 fasting window.
Exercise:
Days 1, 3, 5: 45-minute cardio workout (running, cycling, swimming, etc.).
Days 2, 4, 6: Full-body strength training - 3 sets of 12-15 reps each.

Week 3 - Progression:

Intermittent Fasting (IF): 16/8 method
Days 15-21:
Days 15-21: Maintain the 16/8 fasting window.
Exercise:
Days 1, 3, 5: 30-minute high-intensity interval training (HIIT) session.
Days 2, 4, 6: Upper body and core workout - 3 sets of 12-15 reps each.

Week 4 - Intensification:

Intermittent Fasting (IF): 18/6 method (18 hours fasting, 6 hours eating)
Days 22-28:
Days 22-28: Progress to the 18/6 fasting window.
Exercise:
Days 1, 3, 5: 45-minute cardio or HIIT workout.
Days 2, 4, 6: Lower body and core workout - 3 sets of 12-15 reps each.

Week 5 - Final Push:

Intermittent Fasting (IF): 18/6 method
Days 29-35:
Days 29-35: Continue with the 18/6 fasting window.
Exercise:
Days 1, 3, 5: Full-body circuit training - include a mix of cardio, strength, and flexibility exercises.
Days 2, 4, 6: Active recovery - 30-minute yoga or gentle stretching.
Note: Throughout the 5-week plan, stay hydrated, prioritize whole foods, and include a variety of nutrient-rich options. Monitor your progress, adjust your exercises as needed, and listen to your body. Remember, sustainable weight loss is a gradual process, and consistency is key. Make sure to consult with a healthcare professional or fitness expert before starting any new exercise or diet regimen.

28.

NAVIGATING THE JUNK FOOD JUNGLE: A JOURNEY OF INDULGENCE, INSIGHT, AND EMPOWERMENT

CONCLUSION

As we reach the end of our journey through the world of junk food, indulgence, and culinary exploration, we find ourselves standing at the crossroads of flavor and insight. The pages of this book have taken us on a whirlwind tour of cravings, temptations, cultural influences, and personal transformations. From the allure of empty calories to the captivating tales of junk food redemption, we've explored the multifaceted landscape of our relationship with indulgence. As we conclude this culinary odyssey, we reflect on the lessons learned, the insights gained, and the paths forward toward a balanced and empowered approach to our dietary choices.

Culinary Enlightenment: A Fusion of Knowledge and Taste

Our journey began with a quest for culinary enlightenment, seeking to uncover the hidden truths behind the junk food curtain. We peeled back the layers of marketing strategies, delved into the science of taste, and unraveled the complex web of cravings that often guide our dietary decisions. Along the way, we discovered that the world of junk food is more than just a realm of guilty pleasures – it's a dynamic intersection of culture, psychology, and physiology.

Throughout this exploration, our perspectives have shifted, and we've gained a newfound awareness of the factors that shape our indulgent desires. We've learned to embrace imperfection, celebrate our culinary creativity, and navigate the treacherous terrain of cravings with mindfulness and intention. The tapestry of flavors and insights we've woven together has not only expanded our knowledge but also enriched our culinary experiences.

A Bibliophilic Buffet: References to Other Relevant Books

No culinary journey is complete without a nod to the wisdom shared by other authors who have delved into the intricacies of food, health, and the human palate. Just as we've embarked on a literary feast of indulgence, here are a few other books that provide complementary insights and perspectives on the world of food:

"The Omnivore's Dilemma" by Michael Pollan: A seminal work that delves into the complex web of our modern food system, exploring the origins of our meals and the impact of our dietary choices on health, culture, and the environment.
"Salt, Sugar, Fat" by Michael Moss: Moss takes readers behind the scenes of the processed food industry, revealing how salt, sugar, and fat are meticulously engineered to create addictive and irresistible flavors.
"Mindless Eating" by Brian Wansink: Wansink explores the psychology of eating and

uncovers the subconscious cues that influence our dietary decisions, shedding light on the mindless habits that often lead to overconsumption.

"The End of Overeating" by David A. Kessler: Kessler investigates the science of food addiction, examining how the combination of salt, sugar, and fat in processed foods can create a cycle of overeating and cravings.

"Food Rules" by Michael Pollan: In this concise guide to healthy eating, Pollan offers practical and straightforward principles that can help guide our dietary choices and promote a more mindful and nourishing relationship with food.

These books, along with the insights gathered from our own journey, form a tapestry of knowledge that informs our understanding of the complex interplay between indulgence, health, and culture. Just as a well-prepared meal is a symphony of flavors, these literary works contribute to a rich and nuanced discourse about our relationship with food.

The Road Ahead: Culinary Empowerment and Mindful Balance

As we close the chapter on our exploration of junk food, we stand at the precipice of culinary empowerment and mindful balance. The insights gained from our journey offer us a compass to navigate the ever-evolving landscape of dietary choices. Armed with knowledge, awareness, and a sense of culinary creativity, we can make informed decisions that honor our well-being while still relishing in the occasional indulgence.

Our journey has been one of self-discovery and empowerment, reminding us that our dietary choices are not just a reflection of taste, but also a testament to our values and aspirations. We've learned that embracing imperfection, cultivating mindfulness, and seeking the joy of culinary exploration can lead us toward a more harmonious relationship with food.

As we move forward, let us remember that our culinary choices are not just about what's on our plates – they are a reflection of our connection to ourselves, our communities, and the world around us. By treading mindfully through the junk food jungle, we can savor the flavors of life while honoring our health, values, and the remarkable potential for positive change that lies within each of us.

So, dear reader, may your culinary journey be guided by curiosity, consciousness, and the delight of discovery. As you savor the rich tapestry of flavors that life offers, may you find a sense of empowerment, balance, and joy in every bite.

References:

(Note: The references mentioned here are fictional and provided for illustrative purposes.)

Pollan, M. (2006). The Omnivore's Dilemma: A Natural History of Four Meals. Penguin.
Moss, M. (2013). Salt, Sugar, Fat: How the Food Giants Hooked Us. Random House.
Wansink, B. (2006). Mindless Eating: Why We Eat More Than We Think. Bantam.
Kessler, D. A. (2009). The End of Overeating: Taking Control of the Insatiable American Appetite. Rodale Books.
Pollan, M. (2011). Food Rules: An Eater's Manual. Penguin.

In the pages of this book, we've embarked on a journey through the tantalizing world of junk food, uncovering the mysteries of cravings, exploring the cultural impact of indulgence, and celebrating the stories of redemption and transformation. It has been a culinary expedition that has broadened our horizons, challenged our perspectives, and left us with a deeper understanding of the complex interplay between taste, desire, and conscious consumption. As we bid farewell to the pages that have accompanied us on this journey, we emerge with a newfound sense of empowerment and purpose. Our exploration of the junk food jungle has equipped us with the tools to make informed choices, embrace moderation, and navigate the temptations that surround us.

As we step away from these words and embark on our own culinary adventures, let us carry with us the lessons of mindfulness, balance, and self-awareness. Let us approach each meal as an opportunity to nourish not only our bodies but also our souls. Let us remember that indulgence, when approached with intention, can coexist harmoniously with our pursuit of well-being.

The road ahead is filled with choices – some challenging, others delightful. Yet armed with the insights and wisdom gathered here, we possess the ability to discern, to savor, and to find joy in every aspect of our culinary journey. We have woven a tapestry of knowledge, experiences, and aspirations, and it is up to us to shape it into a narrative of vitality and fulfillment.

So, dear reader, as you take your leave from these pages, may you carry with you the spirit of curiosity, the embrace of moderation, and the conviction that you are the master of your culinary destiny. May your exploration of the junk food jungle be a voyage of empowerment, a celebration of taste, and a testament to the remarkable potential within us all.

Farewell, fellow traveler. May your path be one of mindful choices, delectable pleasures, and a life well-lived through the lens of conscious consumption.

Bon appétit and bon voyage.

ABOUT THE AUTHOR

Umesh Pherwani is a life coach a NLP trainer and a keynote speaker.His first book 'Are you out of your mind' was very well received and marked his first steps into the literary world.
Born in Mumbai, he completed his Masters in Psychology and is pursuing a Ph.D. in the same line of study. Umesh completed a 125 hours

program in neuroscience and the neurobiology of behavior from Stanford university.

His second book was The Mind Switch which was the first in the trio series, followed by The Body Switch and The Gut Switch.

The multi-faceted Umesh is also a model and actor—his most famous show being Family No. 1 on Sony TV. Roll Sound Camera Action, a feature film awaiting release, will see him play the lead. A born entertainer, he is also a stand-up comedian and has performed to houseful shows in Mumbai, Dubai, Abu Dhabi, Bangkok, Amsterdam and St. Martin.

Awards he's won include being bestowed with the title Mr. Popular, which he won as part of the Grasim Mr. India pageant in 2003.

During his spare time, Umesh loves to write and has a food and lifestyle blog.

Umesh loves to take on new challenges, he went on to lose 32 kgs in 3 months after following a strict diet and workout regime.

His second book was The Mind Switch which was the first in the trio series, followed by The Body Switch and The Gut Switch.

Umesh has also authored a fiction novel 'Shadows Embrace' which is a fast faced spy thriller. It is an electrifying tale that explores the complex dynamic of love,duty and sacrifice in the world of espionage.